An Introduction to
Cancer Medicine

An Introduction to Cancer Medicine

KENNETH C. CALMAN
M.D., Ph.D.
Cancer Research Campaign
Professor of Clinical Oncology,
The University of Glasgow, Scotland

and

JOHN PAUL
M.B., Ch.B., Ph.D., F.R.S.E.
Director, Beatson Institute for Cancer Research,
Glasgow, Scotland

A WILEY MEDICAL PUBLICATION
JOHN WILEY & SONS
New York · Chichester · Brisbane · Toronto

John Wiley and Sons Inc.,
605 Third Avenue, New York, NY 10016

First published 1978 by
The Macmillan Press Ltd
London and Basingstoke

© *1978 Kenneth C. Calman and John Paul*

Printed in Hong Kong

Library of Congress Cataloging in Publication Data

Calman, Kenneth Charles.
    An introduction to cancer medicine.

    Bibliography: p.
    Includes index.
    1. Cancer. 2. Cancer education. I. Paul, John,
1922–   joint author. II. Title.
[DNLM: 1. Neoplasms. QZ200 C164i]
RC261. C258   616.9′94   77–91854
ISBN 0-471–04274–9

Contents

Preface

This book has grown out of a number of discussions between clinicians and scientists in an attempt to define the place of cancer medicine in the undergraduate medical curriculum. It is also a reflexion of a new attitude to the approach to cancer by the integration, not only of the basic and clinical aspects of the subject, but of the many clinical disciplines involved in cancer care. It is intended, therefore, as an introduction to the subject for medical students.

However, it is clear that many other professional groups including nurses, social workers and other ancillary workers, together with basic scientists, might welcome such a volume. For this reason some of the sections of the book have been adjusted to meet this need.

During the preparation of this book, many colleagues have been consulted, and we gratefully acknowledge their help and advice. We are indebted for secretarial help to Mrs M. McLeod, Miss E. Dickson, Mrs M. Downie and Mrs J. Peffer, and for artwork to Mr Donald and Mr Ellis. Finally we would like to express our thanks to Mr Charles Fry and the staff of The Macmillan Press for their help in producing this book.

Glasgow, 1977

K.C.C.
J.P.

1 Introduction

Cancer is an emotional word, a word associated with disease, death and dying. It is a word which strikes fear into the hearts of ordinary people because, for centuries, it has been associated with a mysterious illness with no known cause and no known cure. However, during the past 20 years the situation has been transformed; our understanding of the underlying disorder has improved enormously and effective treatments have been evolved for several kinds of cancer.

As a result of these developments attitudes to the management of the disease have been undergoing radical changes. Until quite recently, cancer patients were treated by general physicians and general surgeons. A high proportion still are. With the increasing use of radiotherapy, more and more patients came under the direct care of radiotherapists – and they more and more have become concerned mainly with the treatment of cancer. Since about 1970 a new development has been the emergence of specialists in cancer medicine. The reason for this has been the greatly increased complexity of handling of cancer patients, due to the emergence of effective chemotherapy and the very heavy laboratory service support required for this and for new methods of monitoring the disease process. Accompanying this trend has been an increasing contribution of basic scientific methodology to both the investigation and management of cancer. This has led to the increasing use of the term 'oncology', which is derived from *oncos*, meaning a lump and *logos* meaning study. Hence, oncology is that branch of medical science which deals with the study of tumours. The traditional approaches to the treatment of patients with cancer by the surgeon, physician and radiotherapist are now tending to be called surgical, medical and radiation oncology, particularly in the USA.

Cancer is a common disease. In adults it is second only to diseases of the heart in terms of mortality rates (table 1.1). In childhood it is second only to

Table 1.1   Mortality for leading causes of death (1969, USA). (American Cancer Society)

	%
(1) Diseases of heart	38
(2) Cancer	17
(3) Stroke	10
(4) Accidents	6.1
(5) Influenza and pneumonia	3.6
(6) Diabetes	2.0
(7) Cirrhosis	1.6
(8) Nephritis and nephrosis	0.5
(9) Others	22.2

Table 1.2   Leading causes of death in children 1–14 years. Rate per 100 000 children. (American Cancer Society)

1938		1968	
(1) Accidents	35.8	(1) Accidents	23.3
(2) Pneumonia	27.8	(2) Cancer	6.7
(3) Diarrhoea	12.9	(3) Congenital malformaties	4.3
(4) Tuberculosis	8.9	(4) Influenza	3.7
(5) Appendicitis	8.9	(5) Heart disease	1.1
(6) Heart disease	7.7	(6) Homicide	0.9
(7) Measles	6.8	(7) Stroke	0.7
(8) Diphtheria	6.6	(8) Meningitis	0.7
(9) Influenza	6.2	(9) Gastritis	0.6
(10) Cancer	5.7	(10) Cystic fibrosis	0.6

accidents as a cause of death (table 1.2). This table shows the striking change in the pattern of childhood mortality over the years, largely due to the elimination of infectious diseases as important causes of death.

What is cancer? At the clinical level the word 'cancer' is used to describe a group of diseases with related clinical features which, if untreated, result in death from overgrowth by the cancer cells. These are among the most important diseases of developed countries in which infectious diseases are well controlled. A high proportion of those who die of cancer do so in childhood or at the age of maximum responsibility. Hence, in human social terms it is of very great importance.

At the cellular level cancers are seen as diseases of abnormal cell growth. The normal checks which operate to prevent one tissue overgrowing others are defective and the cancer cells develop abnormalities which enable histological diagnosis to be made.

The fundamental lesions are almost certainly at the molecular level and are due to abnormalities of nucleic acid and protein metabolism; these are being increasingly understood.

Cancer should not be thought of as a single disease. It is akin to the terms 'infectious diseases' or 'arthritis', terms which indicate a group of diseases which are conveniently associated with each other but have different treatments and prognosis. In recognising that cancer is a group of diseases it is implicit that while some kinds are difficult to treat and have poor survival rates, others can be readily treated with excellent long-term results.

Several other terms are commonly used instead of cancer. They include neoplasm, new growth, mitotic lesion and tumour. 'Tumour' is the oldest of these words. It is a latin word meaning a swelling and originally it was used to describe any kind of swelling (including inflammatory swellings). Nowadays it is used as a general term to describe both benign (or simple) and malignant tumours (see p. 3). 'Cancer' is derived from the Greek word for a crab. It is most commonly used to describe malignant growth. The words 'neoplasm' and 'new growth' are euphemisms, commonly used by the medical profession to avoid using the word 'cancer' in front of patients, while 'mitotic lesion' is one of a number of imprecise terms sometimes used for the same purpose.

CLASSIFICATION OF TUMOURS

Tumours are usually classified as simple (or benign) and malignant. Benign tumours tend to remain localised, are often surrounded by a capsule and rarely give rise to serious effects. When they do these are usually caused by pressure on vital organs or by secretion of abnormal amounts of products such as hormones. Malignant tumours, on the other hand, do not remain localised but invade other tissues and give rise to secondary tumours (metastases) in other parts of the body. Malignant tumours commonly cause death by extensive damage to normal tissues. A classical example of a benign tumour is the common wart while cancer of the breast is a classical example of a malignant tumour. This division is operationally convenient and useful both for the pathologist and the clinician but it is by no means clearcut for many benign tumours progress to become malignant. Although the common wart (a papilloma of the skin) almost never becomes malignant, papillomas of the bladder or the colon do so with high frequency.

The progress of a tumour from being benign to becoming malignant sometimes follows quite well-defined stages and, indeed, many tumours have their own natural history. Progressive changes in the evolution of tumours have been charted in experimental animal tumours, particularly rat hepatomas. Some hepatomas in the rat, when first induced, resemble normal tissue very closely indeed; they are described as minimal deviation hepatomas. Morphologically the cells resemble normal hepatocytes but divide at a higher rate and the tissue structure becomes disorganised; consequently, they form distinct tumours. When studied biochemically at this stage, they are often found to contain most of the enzymes associated with normal liver cells but sometimes they show abnormal features. For example, enzymes which can be induced by steroids are no longer inducible. During serial transplantation or culture of these tumours progressive changes occur. Control of other enzymes is progressively lost and eventually some of the enzymes themselves disappear. In due course the result may be a quite anaplastic tumour in which the cells are no longer recognisable as liver cells either morphologically or by biochemical criteria. This phenomenon gave rise to the deletion hypothesis of cancer which proposes, in effect, that cancer is a progressive catastrophe within cells rather than a disorder resulting from a single mutation.

The natural history of many human tumours, although not so carefully studied, follows a very similar pattern. Tissue-specific antigens are progressively lost and tissue-specific functions gradually disappear. Not infrequently, these functional changes are associated with progressive changes in chromosomes.

Tumours are classified in different ways. One of the most general classifications is according to the embryological origin of the tissues (table 1.3). Most benign tumours are described by a word ending in *oma*, such as fibroma. Malignant tumours are generally referred to as sarcomas or carcinomas.

Table 1.3   Classification of the commoner types of tumours

Tissue	Normal cells involved	Benign tumour	Malignant tumour
Connective tissue and muscle	Fibrocyte	Fibroma Myxoma	Fibrosarcoma Myxosarcoma
	Fat cell	Lipoma	Liposarcoma
	Osteocyte	Osteoma	Osteosarcoma
	Muscle	Myoma	Myosarcoma
	Muscle, smooth	Leiomyoma	Leiomyosarcoma
	Muscle, striped	Rhabdomyoma	Rhabdomyosarcoma
Vascular endothelium		Haemangioma Lymphangioma	Haemangiosarcoma
Epithelium	Squamous and transitional	Papilloma	Carcinoma (squamous, basal-cell)
	Glandular	Adenoma	Glandular carcinoma
Neural	Glial	Glioma	
	Nerve	Ganglionic neuroma	Sympathicoblastoma (neuroblastoma)
	Melanoblast	Melanoma	Malignant melanoma Ocular melanoma
Haemopoietic	Reticulum cell	Lymphoma	Lymphosarcoma
	Plasma cell		Reticulosarcoma
	Leucocytes		Myeloma
			Leukaemia
Embryonal		Teratoma	Teratocarcinoma Chorioncarcinoma

MANAGEMENT OF CANCER PATIENTS

Much of this book will be devoted to discussing the special features of treatment of cancer patients. Different varieties of the disease demand different management but there are two principles which may be emphasised here because they put the rest of the book into perspective.

The first is the concept of combined modality therapy. This is the principle of using several methods of treatment on an individual patient. Since many forms of cancer therapy result in profound disturbances of normal body tissues, notably the blood and immune systems, extensive back-up facilities are needed. A multitude of specialities may be involved in the effective treatment of a single cancer patient and the psychological and social disturbances he faces are profound. Hence a team approach is essential.

The second principle naturally follows, that of the cancer-care team composed of doctors, nurses, social workers, physiotherapists, pharmacists, other ancillary workers, the clergy and scientists.

Part 1
Basic Aspects of Cancer

2 The Cancer Cell

Cancer occurs not only in humans but also in other animals and plants. Hence, although we are mainly concerned with it as an affliction which affects us all as sufferers, relatives and friends of sufferers or in the course of our professional responsibilities, it poses many important and challenging questions in biology and, in order to understand it, cancer must be considered in its biological context.

Cancer has been known and recognised as a disease distinct from other causes of swelling for thousands of years but it was only with the discovery of the cell in the seventeenth century, and the emergence of the cell theory a hundred years ago, that a basis for understanding its true nature was established. We now know that it results from the overgrowth, malfunctioning and, sometimes, abnormal migration of some of the cells in multicellular creatures.

An adult human being is made up of about thirty million million individual cells. For comparison, the present population of the world is about four thousand million; hence, there are more than a thousand times as many individual cells in every human being as there are people in the world. Yet, in many ways, cells in an animal behave like individuals in human society. Like human beings, each cell has a dual existence, partly as an individual and partly as a member of a harmoniously functioning community. Knowing the defects of our human society, it is hardly surprising that in the course of fifty years or so some cells in a percentage of people escape from the rules which govern their behaviour and form cancers. It is perhaps more astonishing that cancer does not arise more often. Indeed, it is now believed that the changes which give rise to cancer cells occur more frequently than the incidence of cancer would suggest but that the body has ways of preventing these from giving rise to rogue cells. These will be discussed in chapters 6 and 7.

CELL STRUCTURE AND FUNCTION

Although our bodies contain many different kinds of cells, they are all built to the same general plan with a limited set of components. We can, therefore, describe cells in terms of a 'typical' cell (figure 2.1) based on the appearance of a simple fibroblast or epithelial cell as seen in tissue culture. Differentiated cells can be distinguished by the ways in which they differ from this typical cell. Not all cells in a human are alike but they are all essential components of the individual and normally work together in a perfectly harmonious relationship. This entails rigorous regulation of the growth, migration and specialised functions of cells. If taken out of the body and grown in tissue culture, they behave quite differently. Then, most cells reveal that they are capable of quite rapid growth and can migrate freely; these functions must, therefore, be kept constantly in check within our bodies. In other words, cells

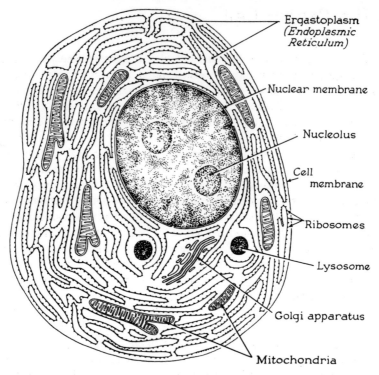

Figure 2.1   Diagram of a 'typical' animal cell. (Paul, J., *Cell and Tissue Culture*, Livingstone, London, 1959)

exhibit what has been appropriately called social behaviour, exemplified by the facts that they remain localised in appropriate organs and the rate of cell division is restricted to that required to maintain the proper size of each organ. Liver cells are never found outside the liver and usually show a very low rate of cell division, just sufficient to replace cells which accidentally die. However, if a part of the liver is removed, the remaining cells rapidly multiply until the deficiency has been restored. They then revert to the slow division rate. Cancer is a disease of cells which results in their growing when they should not, migrating to tissues where they should not normally be and performing functions other than those which they would normally be expected to perform.

CELL MEMBRANE

The cell is enclosed in a cell membrane composed of lipid and protein molecules, the basic structure of which is a double layer of lipid molecules. It has a semifluid character and, being lipid, restricts the passage of water molecules and water soluble molecules between the inside of the cell and the outside. If it were solely a lipid membrane, it would be very highly impermeable indeed to these kinds of molecules and this would not be compatible with survival since most of the nutrients which cells require are water soluble. However, the properties of the lipid membrane are modified by the presence of proteins within it. Some of these are confined to the outside of the membrane and some to the inside but some pass completely through it (figure 2.2). Some are enzymes and others enzyme-like proteins which facilitate the passage of special molecules in and out of the cell. For example, one kind provides a special transport mechanism for calcium ions but probably for no others while yet another may act as a transportation mechanism for phosphate.

It is at the same membrane that the cell encounters its external environment and while this may vary, the interior of the cell has to be kept relatively constant. Thus, the membrane is not simply a passive envelope but an active organelle responsible for maintaining the internal environment. Not surprisingly, we find that certain specific stimuli, notably hormones, have their primary actions on the cell membrane. For example, insulin influences the permeability of the membrane to glucose and other hormones activate the adenyl cyclases located at the membrane.

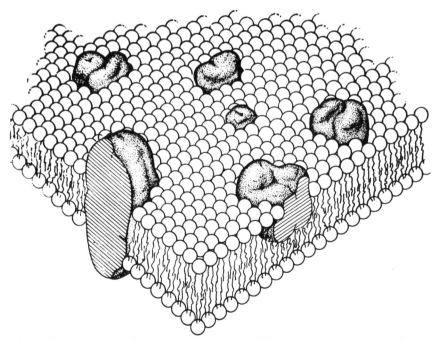

Figure 2.2   Structure of the cell membrane. Lipid molecules are represented by spheres with tails. These form a double membrane. The irregular shapes embedded in the membrane and, in one case, passing through it, represent integral globular proteins. (Singer, S. J. and Nicolson, G. L., *Science*, **175**, 723, 1972)

The membrane is rarely, if ever, completely naked but has a protective coating around it, the cell wall. In plant cells, this is very prominent and consists of the celluloses and lignins which are typical of plant tissues. The cell wall in animals is less prominent but has many similarities to plant cell walls. In particular, it contains mucopolysaccharides. They are antigenic; antibodies against living cells usually react with them and are commonly cell-specific. 'Cell surface antigens' are important in tumour immunology as discussed in chapter 7. It is quite likely that they are concerned with cell recognition, the ability of a cell to recognise whether an adjacent cell is similar or different. This property may provide signals between cells; therefore, it may be important in the control of cell migration.

THE NUCLEUS

The most prominent structure within a cell is the nucleus which is the repository of genetic information stored with the chromosomes. It is separated from the cytoplasm by a double membrane, similar in structure to the cell membrane except that it has holes, nuclear pores, which establish communications between nucleus and cytoplasm. Chromosomes are not visible most of the time and only become obvious during the mitotic stage of the cell cycle. At any time, most cells are in a stage of the cell-cycle called interphase, during which the material of the chromosomes, called chromatin, takes the form of very long threads coiled like skeins of wool. In some parts of the nucleus, the chromatin is rather condensed and in other places, relatively uncondensed. The condensed chromatin is referred to as heterochromatin and the uncondensed material as euchromatin. The nucleolus is a particularly dense spherical structure within the nucleus; it is sometimes double or multiple and can usually be easily recognised.

CYTOPLASMIC STRUCTURES

In the cytoplasm, there are several other distinctive structures (figure 2.3). *Mitochondria* vary in shape but are usually sausage-shaped and in electron microscope sections can be seen to have inner folds, called cristae (figure 2.3). They have been very extensively studied and are known to be the structures in which most of the reactions of cellular respiration occur. They are involved in the oxidative breakdown of carbohydrate and lipid molecules and with storage of the released energy as adenosinetriphosphate (ATP), which is used for most of the energy requiring processes of the cell. Because of these functions, the mitochondrion is sometimes referred to as the powerhouse of the cell.

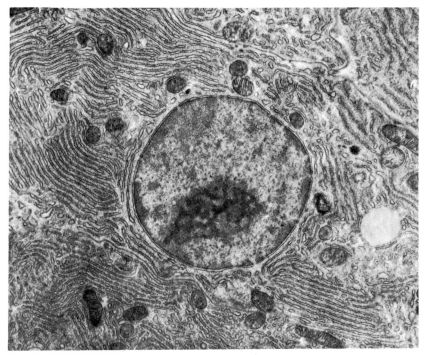

Figure 2.3   Electron microscopic section of a pancreatic acinar cell. (Dr D. Fawcett)

In electron micrographs, other, rather solid, spherical structures about the same size as mitochondria can be seen. There are at least two kinds, *lysosomes* and *peroxisomes*, both being involved in digestive processes. The lysosomes are membrane-enclosed bags containing enzymes such as proteases and nucleases which break down proteins and nucleic acids respectively. The peroxisomes contain some specialised oxidising enzymes. Most cells, but particularly scavenger types of cells, can engulf food by an invagination and sealing off of portions of the cell membrane, a process called pinocytosis. The result is the formation within the cytoplasm of vacuoles containing the fluids in which the cell is bathed. Lysosomes fuse with these vacuoles and discharge their digestive enzymes into them (figure 2.4). In this way, large molecules are broken down into small molecules which can diffuse through the membrane into the cytoplasm to be metabolised by the cell's biochemical machinery.

There is one other major membrane-associated system within the cytoplasm, the *endoplasmic reticulum* and the *Golgi apparatus*. The endoplasmic reticulum consists of a series of folded and packed membranes similar to a plastic bag from which most of the air has been withdrawn. Some parts of the membrane are smooth but much of it is studded with ribosomes. These are involved in the synthesis of proteins which accumulate inside the

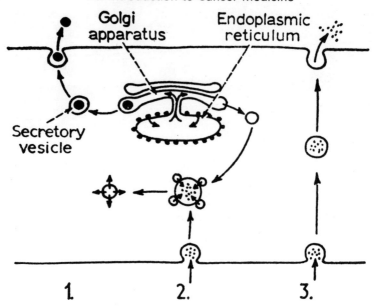

Figure 2.4   Secretion, pinocytosis and lysosomes. Spheres containing proteins to be secreted by the cells are formed by nipping off small portions of the Golgi apparatus as in 1. Substances in the environment may be taken into the cell by pinocytosis as in 2. Lysosomes fuse with these to form digestive vacuoles as in 2. Sometimes pinocytic vacuoles can pass through a cell and release their products on the other side as in 3.
(Paul, J., *Cell Biology*, 2nd ed., Heinemann, London, 1967)

bag. The Golgi apparatus is a specially modified region of this structure in which newly synthesised proteins accumulate. In cells with secretory functions, portions of the Golgi apparatus become nipped off to form secretory droplets which pass to the surface of the cell where they burst, discharging their contents into the surrounding fluid.

Electron micrographs reveal that many cells also have a system of filaments and tubules running through them. The filaments probably form a structural framework for the cell. The microtubules appear to be associated mainly with contractile functions; they form a prominent component of cilia, the threadlike structures on the surface of some epithelial cells which beat rhythmically and move substances over their surfaces.

During cell division, the *mitotic spindle* appears. This is composed of microtubules and is concerned with the segregation of the chromosomes. Spindles have their origin in *centrioles* which are visible in interphase as well as during mitosis.

Granules, about ten nanometres in diameter, called ribosomes, are a prominent feature of the cytoplasm. As already mentioned, in secretory cells with an extensive endoplasmic reticulum they are often distributed densely along it in clusters of four or five or more, called polysomes. In other cells, polysomes are free in the cytoplasm. These structures are concerned with protein synthesis.

INFORMATION FLOW AND PROTEIN SYNTHESIS

All metabolic processes are carried out by enzymes. These are proteins as are also most of the structural components of cells. Hence, both functional and structural characteristics of cells are determined mainly by the range of proteins they contain and protein synthesis is the most basic of all life processes. The proteins themselves are synthesised in polysomes but the information for this process is encoded in the DNA in the chromosomes in the nucleus.

Every cell in the body contains the same DNA which carries instructions

Table 2.1   The genetic code. A: adenosine, C: cytosine, G: guanine, U: uracil

Amino acid	Common bases	Code triplets (codons) Complete triplets			
Phenylalanine	UU—	UUU	UUC		
Leucine	UU—			UUA	UUG
	CU—	CUU	CUC	CUA	CUG
Isoleucine	AU—	AUU	AUC	AUA	
Methionine	AU—				AUG
Valine	GU—	GUU	GUC	GUA	GUG
Serine (1)	UC—	UCU	UCC	UCA	UCG
Proline	CC—	CCU	CCC	CCA	CCG
Threonine	AC—	ACU	ACC	ACA	ACG
Alanine	GC—	GCU	GCC	GCA	GCG
Tyrosine	UA—	UAU	UAC		
End of message	UA—			UAA	UAG
Histidine	CA—	CAU	CAC		
Glutamine	CA—			CAA	CAG
Asparagine	AA—	AAU	AAC		
Lysine	AA—			AAA	AAG
Aspartic acid	GA—	GAU	GAC		
Glutamic acid	GA—			GAA	GAG
Cysteine	UG—	UGU	UGC		
Tryptophan	UG—				UGG
Arginine	CG—	CGU	CGC	CGA	CGG
	AG—			AGA	AGG
Serine, (2)	AG—	AGU	AGC		
Glycine	GG—	GGU	GGC	GGA	GGG

for all cell components. The difference between a liver cell and a brain cell is not in the genetic information it contains but in the genetic information it uses.

DNA (deoxyribonucleic acid) is made up of four component nucleotides, deoxyadenylic acid (A), deoxythymidylic acid (T), deoxycytidylic acid (C) and deoxyguanylic acid (G) (figure 2.5). These four nucleotides form the four

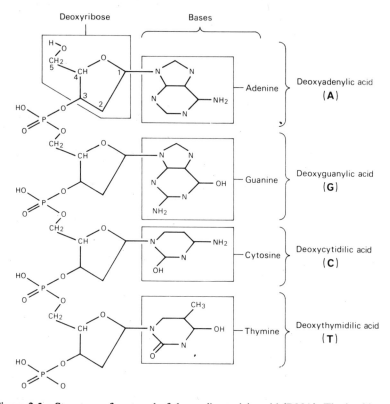

Figure 2.5   Structure of a strand of deoxyribonucleic acid (DNA). The backbone is formed by a chain of deoxyribose molecules linked together through phosphate groups. To each deoxyribose molecule is linked one of four organic bases. Adenine and guanine are purine bases, cytosine and thymine are pyrimidine bases. The combination of a base, a deoxyribose molecule and a phosphate molecule comprise a nucleotide such as deoxyadenylic acid. The sequence of nucleotides forms the code which carries genetic information

signals in the genetic code which is analogous to the morse code. Just as the combination of signals in the morse code can code for the 26 letters of our alphabet, combinations of the four nucleotides in the genetic code, in groups of three, code for the 20 amino acids which make up nearly all known proteins (table 2.1). Just as an encyclopaedia could be written in morse code,

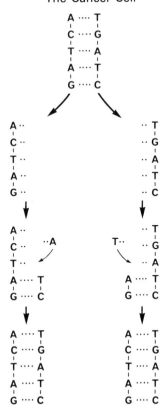

Figure 2.6   The way in which two strands of DNA interact, by hydrogen bonds, to form a double-stranded DNA molecule (top). When the DNA molecule replicates it first separates into two single strands. The enzyme DNA polymerase then builds up a complementary strand to each of these by stitching together free nucleotides. In this way, two identical double-stranded molecules are formed (bottom)

so the amino acid sequence of all known proteins can be written in the genetic code.

Hence, the information for the amino acid sequences for all the proteins in a human being is deposited in the DNA in the nucleus of every cell. DNA is a double-stranded structure. The information for protein is encoded in the 'sense strand' of DNA; this is paired with another strand, the 'nonsense' strand, which is related to it as a photographic negative is related to a photographic positive. This relationship is established by the fact that an A in one strand is always opposite a T in the other and a C in one strand is always opposite a G in the other (figure 2.6). This arrangement is necessary for replication of DNA.

Since genetic information resides in the nucleus but proteins are made in polysomes in the cytoplasm, there has to be some mechanism for conveying information from nucleus to cytoplasm (figure 2.7). First an RNA copy of the

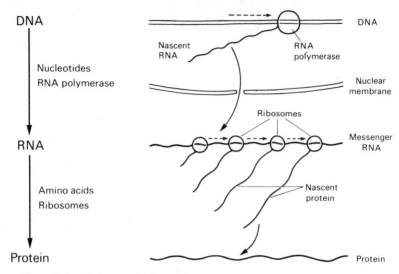

Figure 2.7　Pathway of information transport from nucleus to cytoplasm

DNA of a gene, messenger RNA, is made; this bears the same relationship to the sense strand of DNA as a negative to a positive photograph. The messenger RNA molecule passes from the chromosomes in the nucleus to the polysomes in the cytoplasm taking information for protein synthesis with it. Some of the differences between diferent cells are achieved by a kind of selection mechanism, so far not fully understood, which results in copies being prepared from certain parts of the DNA and not from other parts.

When the messenger RNA enters the cytoplasm, it becomes associated with some other molecules which participate with it in a cycle of protein synthesis. A ribosome first becomes attached to the beginning of the message and passes along it reading it or translating it as it does so by taking up amino acids from the medium and stitching them together in the correct sequence, according to the instructions in the messenger RNA. The amino acids in the cytoplasm do not float around; they are attached to transfer RNA molecules which function as adaptors and bring the amino acids into the right relationship to each other, according to the information encoded in the messenger RNA molecule.

Usually more than one ribosome is at work on a messenger RNA molecule at any one time and a polysome is made up of a group of ribosomes attached to a single messenger.

ENERGY METABOLISM

Most of the energy required by cells is obtained by oxidising carbohydrates or lipids. The overall effect is the consumption of oxygen, the formation of carbon dioxide and water and the synthesis of 'high energy phosphate bonds'. The best known of the high energy phosphate bonds is that which is formed when inorganic phosphate is attached to adenosine diphosphate (ADP) to form adenosine triphosphate (ATP). The formation of this bond requires a considerable amount of energy and when the bond is broken that energy is released and can be used in metabolic processes. ATP can be synthesised in the cell in many ways but three metabolic pathways are particularly important. The first is called anaerobic glycolysis. As its name implies, this does not involve the uptake of oxygen. It results in the formation of lactic acid at the expense of glucose with the formation of some ATP. It is not a very efficient process but it is quite important in cancer cells since there is much evidence that cancer cells use this particular energy pathway more than most other cells in the body. The other two pathways are both oxidative pathways. The most important is the Krebs cycle in which pyruvic acid, formed by glycolysis, is oxidised to form carbon dioxide, water and a large amount of ATP. This is the main source of ATP in most cells and most of this process is carried on in mitochondria. There is another important pathway called the pentose shunt which also results in the breakdown of glucose to carbon dioxide and water, with the synthesis of a large number of high energy bonds; but its main functions are probably to produce some of the molecules needed to make nucleic acids and some used in other synthetic processes.

CELL DIFFERENTIATION

In normal development, the fertilised egg cell at first divides very rapidly. A small group of cells is formed in which the individual cells are apparently identical and then, at a very early stage, differences appear among them. Within two or three weeks, an embryo has emerged with clearly different tissues such as blood and muscle. Since all the cells in different tissues have exactly the same kind of genetic information, why are the cells different? We do not fully understand the reasons but it seems that divergences arise as a result of controls at different stages in the synthesis of proteins. Some arise when messenger RNA is being made from DNA; in certain cells some genes are copied but others are not, while in other cells different sets of genes may be copied. In each cell, some thousands of genes, possibly tens of thousands, are in use at any one time. Differences can occur in the use of messenger RNA at other levels of protein synthesis too.

As an example of these mechanisms, the development of red blood cells is instructive. The genes which give rise to the globin chains of haemoglobin are transcribed at a high rate in blood-forming cells but may not be transcribed at all in other kinds of cells such as brain cells. At different stages of foetal development, different kinds of haemoglobin are made (for example, foetal and adult haemoglobin) and, therefore, different globin genes are switched on during different stages of development. This switching is done in a very orderly fashion like the switching processes in a computer.

These processes, by means of which different cells are caused to specialise, are obviously very important to cancer because it is almost certainly a disturbance of these mechanisms which gives rise to the abnormalities which characterise the cancer cell. Unfortunately, however, we do not yet understand them fully.

CELL DIVISION

If left to grow freely, many animal cells will divide every twelve to twenty-four hours. During the greater part of this time, very little seems to happen when viewed with the microscope except that the cell becomes progressively larger. When it has doubled in volume, it suddenly enters into mitosis and then dramatic morphological changes take place (figure 2.8). The nucleus begins to break up and the chromosomes form. These progressively condense and line up across the middle of the cell in the metaphase plate. They then sort themselves out into two identical sets, each of which goes to a different end of the cell. Finally, the cell is nipped into two cells with one set of chromosomes in each.

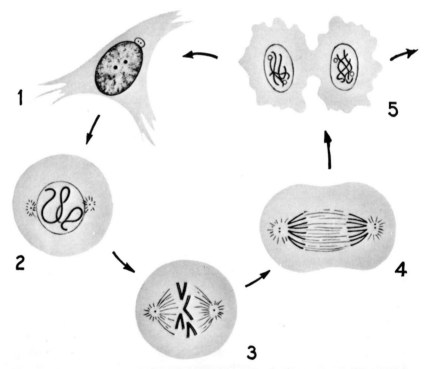

Figure 2.8   Main stages during mitosis: (1) interphase; (2) prophase; (3) metaphase; (4) anaphase; (5) telophase. (Paul, J., *Cell and Tissue Culture*, Livingstone, London, 1959)

When observed with the microscope, all the interesting events seem to happen during the brief period of an hour or so during which mitosis occurs. However, appearances are misleading and, in fact, during the rest of the cell cycle (called interphase) some most important metabolic events occur. During this time all the molecules in a cell have to be duplicated to make enough material for two cells. A particularly important event is the synthesis of new DNA and the duplication of the chromosomes. In this process, the two strands of the DNA molecule unzip like a zip fastener. Each half then creates a new half in the mirror image of itself by accumulating nucleotides, A pairing with T, G pairing with C, and, in this way, two new sets of genetic information arise, providing the material for two identical sets of chromosomes (figure 2.6).

This process does not occur continually during interphase but takes place in a specific period of about four or five hours called the S (DNA synthesis) phase. The S phase occurs roughly in the middle of interphase and helps to divide it into three parts. The period preceding S, between the previous mitosis and the beginning of S phase, is called G_1 (the first gap) and the time between the end of DNA synthesis and the commencement of mitosis is called G_2 (the second gap). Proteins and other cellular components are made throughout the cell cycle but in the G_1 phase these include proteins needed for replication of the chromatin while in the G_2 phase they include some of the proteins required for mitosis.

In a suitable medium, if growth is unrestricted, cells will go on dividing day after day. The consequences of completely unrestricted growth are interesting to contemplate. If cells divide once a day, then, starting on the first day with one cell, we would have two cells the following day, four cells the next day, eight cells the next day and so on. After about one month, the cells would have undergone approximately thirty divisions, yielding about one thousand million cells, weighing one or two grams. This is the rate at which cells grow in the earliest stages of embryonic development. Now, if this rate of growth were maintained for a second month, and all the cells and their progeny were retained during that time, we would find ourselves with two or three hundred thousand kilograms of cells! In less than a year, the universe would be packed solid with cells. This, of course, is an absurd idea but it illustrates very clearly that uncontrolled cell growth almost never occurs and when it does, it lasts for a very short time.

The rate at which a population of cells grows is, in fact, controlled by a number of factors, some specific and some non-specific. The first is the cell cycle time of the cell, the time taken to pass from a fixed point in the cell cycle, say mitosis, to the same fixed point in the next cell cycle. This is characteristic of the cell type itself. In the earliest stages of development in mammals, the cell cycle may be as short as 8–10 hours. Some of the blood-forming cells in the bone marrow may also divide as quickly as this. On the other hand, some other cells may take several days to complete a cell cycle even when growing at the maximum rate.

Many cells which are capable of very rapid division either do not divide in adult animals or do so very slowly. A striking example is liver cells which in the normal adult exhibit virtually no mitotic activity. However, if a large part of the liver is ablated, by surgery, poisoning or infection (as in acute hepatitis), the remaining normal liver cells divide very rapidly and, in a matter of days, restore the lost tissue. The prolonged resting state of differentiated cells is considered by some to represent a very extended G_1 phase but it is usually considered as a special phase called G_0, which provides an alternative to G_1 and requires a special stimulus to cause the cells to return to G_1. The factors which determine whether cells remain in G_0 or go into mitosis may be very important in relation to the mechanism of carcinogenesis but they are not understood.

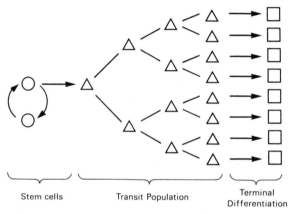

Stem cells   Transit Population   Terminal Differentiation

Figure 2.9   Relationship of differentiated cells to stem cells, illustrating amplification of cell number by a transit population

Some cells in the body do behave like those described above in that each cell, on dividing, gives rise to two identical daughter cells. However, in many tissues cell lineages behave quite differently in that stem cells give rise to non-identical daughters, one of which is destined to form more stem cells and the other of which is destined to differentiate into a mature, often non-dividing, differentiated cell (figure 2.9). The most thoroughly studied example of such a population in the human is blood formation. Here we know that there is a population of stem cells, each capable of giving rise to most of the different types of cells in blood. This population divides quite slowly and its progeny have two functions. On the one hand, they have to maintain the size of the stem cell population itself and, on the other, they have to give rise to all the differentiated cells such as erythrocytes, platelets and granulocytes. From the behaviour of these cells in the animal, we know that they respond to the requirements of the organism. If more stem cells are needed, more stem cells are produced. If more red cells are needed, more red cells are produced. At present there is only a very rudimentary understanding of these regulatory factors but, clearly, knowledge of them would be of very great importance in understanding cancer, since cancer cells often fail to respond to the correct control signals. In connection with stem cell populations, it is worth while pointing out that the differentiated cells arising from stem cells very often are incapable of division (for example, erythrocytes). Hence, this kind of population does not grow exponentially like the growing cells referred to earlier.

Within stem cell type populations, there very often occurs another group of cells forming a dividing transit population (figure 2.9). Again, a good example is in erythropoiesis. It is known that each stem cell may given rise to a very large number, perhaps several hundred, red cells and so there has to be some amplification of cell number during the differentiation from stem cell to red cell. This occurs in cells, committed erythroid precursors, which are descendants from the original stem cell, though not themselves stem cells, and which will give rise to mature red cells, though not themselves mature red cells. Within the compartment cells multiply rapidly in much the same way as the exponential population described above. The difference is that cells are constantly being fed into this population and removed from it so that the size of the transit population remains more or less constant.

Tumour cells, especially in the more differentiated cancers, often behave in the same manner. Mitosis may be confined to one fraction, termed the growth fraction, corresponding to the transit population of erythropoietic cells. The non-growing fraction is recognised as comprising two populations: one, incapable of further division, termed the non-clonogenic fraction and the other, termed the clonogenic fraction, composed of cells in G_0 which can re-enter mitosis and give rise to a new growth fraction.

The intrinsic patterns of growth which have been described are profoundly affected by environmental factors. An obvious example is the availability of nutritional substances from the tissue fluids. The extent to which this restricts normal growth is not known but it certainly plays an important part in the growth of tumour cells. It is a common feature of solid tumours that they are necrotic in the centre, due to the fact that the tumour cells outgrow their blood supply. Obviously the cells nearest a good blood supply grow fastest while those further away are likely to grow slower because of limitation of nutrients. Those furthest away may die for this reason. In a tumour, the overall rate of growth depends on the relative rates of cell division and cell death. When cell division exceeds cell death, the tumour grows, when the two are in balance, the tumour stays stationary and if cell death exceeds cell growth, the tumour regresses. The object of all cancer therapy is to swing this balance in favour of regression. During the early stages, a tumour may grow in an exponential fashion until limitation of nutrients or other factors cause a reduction in growth rate, often accompanied by increased cell-death (figure 2.10). As this figure illustrates, a great number of cell generations may have passed before a tumour is detectable and then relatively few before its growth causes death.

These considerations of tumour cell growth are of great importance in

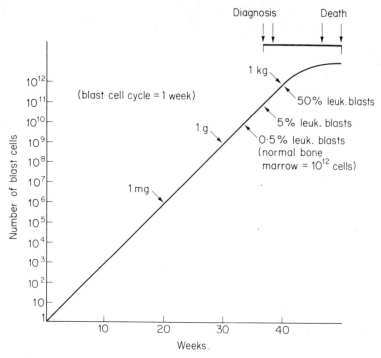

Figure 2.10   Growth of a theoretical leukaemic blast cell population. More than 40 population doublings are required before leukaemia can be properly diagnosed. (Lajtha, L. G. in *What We Know About Cancer* (Ed. R. J. C. Harris), Allen and Unwin, London, 1970, p. 47)

radiotherapy and especially in chemotherapy. They will be referred to in these contexts in chapters 13 and 14.

Besides non-specific factors, growth of cells in the animal is dependent on some specific factors. Certain tissues are hormone-dependent in that their growth depends on availability of the appropriate hormones. The sex organs are well-known examples and this principle is exploited in cancer therapy. For example, the growth of cancer of the breast is reduced, and occasionally regression occurs, if the ovaries are removed. If tumour cells remained hormone-dependent, this would greatly facilitate the treatment of many kinds of cancer. Unfortunately, it is a feature of cancer cells that they tend progressively to escape from hormone-dependence.

There are also less well-understood regulatory factors which are involved in the maintenance of organ size, e.g. as mentioned earlier in relation to liver regeneration. The factors involved in such control have been called 'chalones'. Their nature has not been clearly established but they are thought of as substances produced by cells, which inhibit multiplication of their own kind very specifically. It is postulated that an escape from controls of this kind is an important feature of cancer.

Finally, in relation to growth regulation, another phenomenon has to be mentioned. When certain cells, for example skin cells, come into contact they inhibit each other from moving, a phenomenon called 'contact inhibition'. If the density of cells is reduced they begin to move round again and this is usually correlated with an increase in the rate of mitosis. Very little is known about this phenomenon but, again, it is clearly one of the normal control systems within the body which maintains the normal coordination of function and which is probably defective in many cancers.

CHARACTERISTICS OF CANCER CELLS

Cancer cells have all the structural features of a general cell. It is only when one compares the structure of cancer cells with the special features of the specialised cells of the tissue from which they arise that one recognises obvious anomalies, some of which will be discussed in detail in later chapters. In general, these can be summarised as representing abnormalities of cell differentiation. The structural abnormalities reflect abnormalities in the utilisation of genetic information as a consequence of which the range of proteins within the cancer cell differs from the range of proteins in the cell of origin. One aspect of this is the disappearance of some of the enzymes characteristic of particular tissues. This has been particularly studied in experimental hepatomas (tumours of the liver). Most of these exhibit the absence of several typical liver enzymes and, as the tumours progress, more and more enzymes seem to be missing. On the other side of the coin, tumour cells sometimes produce proteins which they would not normally be expected to produce. A well-known example is the production of ectopic hormones, e.g. pituitary hormones, by some lung tumours. So far as is known none of the cells in the lung ever produce these and this is, therefore, an acquired function. We have to interpret these gains and losses of proteins as representing a profound disturbance in the machinery involved in the expression of genetic information. Some examples of clinical interest are listed in table 2.2.

Another characteristic anomaly of cancer cells is their failure to respond to the normal growth-restraining signals in the body. This has already been mentioned in the discussion of growth. It is, of course, the reason for the most characteristic of all the features of cancer, the production of a swelling (which is the literal translation of the Latin word *tumor*). These changes in response to growth signals are presumably due to changes in the utilisation of genetic information in cells.

The third characteristic of cancer cells is their failure to respond to positional signals in the body. It is well established that most cells, while free to migrate in tissue culture, do not normally do so in the animal. This seems to be because they recognise signals in the environment which tell them when they are in the correct location. Cancer cells, especially malignant cells, are defective in these recognition signals and, therefore, can become established in other tissue.

Table 2.2   Ectopic production of proteins by some tumours

Abnormal protein	Tumour
Erythropoietin	Cerebellar haemangioblastoma, uterine fibroma, hepatoma, (melanoma?)
Adrenocorticotrophic hormone	Bronchogenic carcinoma, thymoma
'Insulin-like' activity	Mesenchymoma
Parathormone	Bronchogenic carcinoma
Thyrotrophin	Trophoblastic tumours
Carcino-embryonic antigen	Carcinoma of colon plus many other tumours
Alpha-fetoprotein	Hepatoma

CELL TRANSFORMATION

Although cells from a far-advanced tumour are often easy to distinguish from normal cells, sometimes the distinction is very difficult indeed to make; one of the most difficult problems in cancer research is simply distinguishing between normal and cancer cells. One way to do this is to inoculate the cells into a suitable host animal. Mouse cells can be inoculated into other mice with an identical genetic constitution to the donor (syngeneic animals). If they form tumours then it is quite certain that they are tumour cells. If they do not form tumours, this can be for a variety of reasons. In particular, the host may not be able to tolerate these cells from the immunological point of view, a subject which will be discussed later. The sensitivity of these experiments is therefore very often increased by suppressing the host's immunological mechanisms.

One reason for wishing to distinguish clearly between cancer and non-cancer cells is to permit studies of the event which results in a normal cell being transformed to a cancer cell. Hence, it would be particularly valuable if this distinction could be made outside the animal, for example, in tissue culture. Such an assay has been developed in which a sudden change or 'transformation' of apparently normal cells occurs (figure 2.11(a) and (b)). Many of the features of transformed cells resemble those of cancer cells. Indeed, cells transformed in tissue culture can often be shown to produce cancers in experimental animals although it is not certain that tissue culture transformation and malignant transformation are exactly the same thing.

The transformation assay depends on the ability to grow, in tissue culture, cells which behave much like normal cells. One kind of cell used in this way is the fibroblast which, when grown in tissue culture, exhibits a characteristic morphology, tending to line up in a parallel arrangement which might be

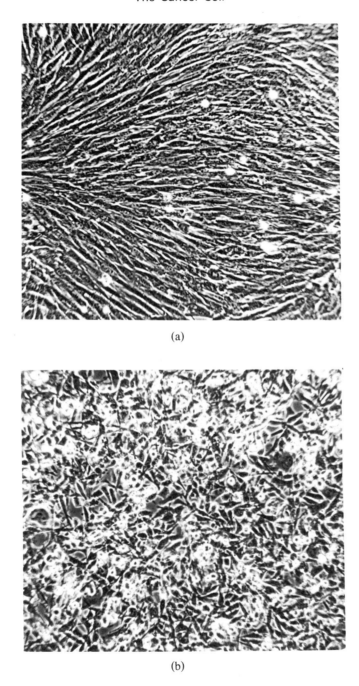

(a)

(b)

Figure 2.11   (a) Normal BHK21 cells showing characteristic parallel alignment; (b) the same cells transformed by polyoma virus (Dr M. G. P. Stoker)

likened to matches in a matchbox (figure 2.11(a)). If cells of this kind are treated with certain tumour viruses, they behave quite differently in that they no longer line up in this orderly manner but grow higgledy-piggledy over each other (figure 2.11(b)) as if the box of matches had been emptied out on to a table. These transformed cells have other characteristics which distinguish them from untransformed fibroblasts. For example, they will grow readily in suspension in some media in which the normal cells will not grow and their surface properties seem to be altered quite specifically. Changes of this kind can be produced by tumour viruses and also by chemicals and other factors which cause cancer, for example irradiation, as discussed in chapter 4.

3 Prevalence of Cancer – Epidemiology

COSTS AND GENERAL INCIDENCE

Since the beginning of this century, the incidence of cancer has increased enormously; the percentage of all deaths attributable to cancer has gone up between four and five times. In Britain, 40 per cent of all cancer deaths in men occur in the 45–60 age group; in women, 40 per cent occur before 55. Hence, many cancer victims are people with social responsibilities and, indeed, in these age groups cancer is a more frequent cause of death than arteriosclerosis. Moreover, the financial cost of cancer is enormous, for example, in 1972, cancer cases in Britain accounted for 5 per cent of all hospital admissions. It was estimated that in that year it cost the Health Service £70 million and that the additional cost to the country was about £500 million. Very similar figures apply to all the developed countries. However, some cancers are much commoner than others and the pattern varies from country to country and from time to time. The variations provide important information and they will form the subject of this chapter. The incidence of the commonest cancers in the USA are shown in table 3.1, from which can be gleaned some estimate of the frequency with which these conditions are likely to be encountered, bearing in mind that the average general practitioner may see a dozen or so cases of cancer each year. Throughout this book, and especially in the next few chapters, dealing with basic aspects of cancer research, many of the examples are of very rare conditions. Because of unique features, these provide valuable information about cancer but it should be understood that many of them will never be seen in the average hospital ward.

Epidemiology is the study of the distribution of disease in different groups of people. Its main aims are (1) to identify, by population studies, causative agents, (2) to identify high risk populations and (3) to describe changes in incidence and mortality. If cancer simply arose in a random manner, it would be more or less evenly distributed throughout the population. There would be occasional coincidences of the sort that occur when a coin is tossed and comes down heads ten times in succession. It is possible mathematically to make allowances for coincidences of this kind and when these are excluded, it very often proves to be the case that, indeed, no particular local variation can be recognised in the occurrence of many forms of cancer. However, not uncommonly, epidemiological studies reveal an abnormal concentration of cases of one kind of cancer in a particular group of people. This is called clustering and when it is observed, it immediately initiates a search for factors which may be responsible for it. The correlation between the distribution of the disease and some other factor does not necessarily prove that that factor is the cause but it frequently provides important clues.

Table 3.1   Age-adjusted incidence rates for 1969 per 100 000 population in USA. (American Cancer Society)

Site	Male	Female
Total	344.5	308.6
Lung and bronchus	70.2	13.2
Uterus	—	76.5
Breast	0.7	74.6
Colon	34.4	29.8
Prostate	58.7	—
Rectum	17.3	11.0
Bladder	22.0	6.0
Lymphomas	15.7	9.8
Stomach	15.9	7.1
Pancreas	12.1	7.4
Leukemias	12.2	7.3
Lip, tongue and mouth	10.8	4.4
Ovary	—	13.9
Eye and nervous system	6.7	5.3
Kidney	7.9	3.9
Larynx	9.1	1.1
Oesophagus	5.7	1.6
Thyroid	2.1	5.0
Pharynx	5.2	1.5
Melanomas–skin	3.2	3.3
Gallbladder and ducts	2.5	3.2
Liver	3.5	1.4
Soft tissues	2.3	1.8
Testis and penis	3.9	—
Bones and joints	1.2	0.8
Other and unspecified sites	21.2	18.7

Sometimes clustering is geographical, suggesting that an environmental factor is involved, sometimes it occurs in a particular occupational group and this stimulates a search for a carcinogenic factor associated with the occupation. In many cases, several factors can be correlated with the high frequency of the disease and the researcher is then faced with the challenge of identifying the critical one.

In some cancers, the clustering is so obvious that it is unnecessary to employ sophisticated statistical methods to detect it. Some of the earliest observations on the causes of cancer arose simply because physicians were able to observe that certain groups of people exhibited a particularly high prevalence of certain kinds of cancer. One of the first observations of this kind was made in Padua in the year 1700 by the physician Bernardino Ramazzini who reported that there was a higher incidence of mammary cancer in nuns than in the general population. This observation was verified by another Italian, Domenico Antonio Rigoni-Stern, who studied the causes of death in Verona between the years 1760 and 1839 and found that cancer of the breast was five times more frequent among nuns than among other women. He reported these findings in 1844.

The best known observation of this nature was that made by Percival Pott, a London surgeon, who published in 1775 a description of cancer of the scrotum in chimney sweeps. Although Pott was the first to report the relationship between exposure to soot and the occurrence of cancer, he was not the first to make the observation because he himself remarked that, in the trade, cancer of the scrotum of this nature was referred to as the soot wart. It took another 150 years before the Japanese scientists Yamagiwa and Ichikawa showed, by painting coal tar on rabbit skin, that this was a direct cause of skin cancer. This observation eventually led to the isolation of the pure chemical carcinogen, benzpyrine, by Kennaway's group in 1930.

Another early report of an occupational cancer related to the high incidence of lung cancer in miners in Schneeberg in Austria. These tumours were probably caused by the inhalation of uranium dust and although they were not reported as being related to the occupation of the miners until the late 19th century, the occurrence of lung disease among the miners was common knowledge in the region for hundreds of years before that.

With these classical examples before them, physicians of the late 19th and early 20th century became more and more alert to the possible relationship between environmental circumstances and the occurrence of particular kinds of cancer. Rehn, for example, reported that bladder cancer was exceptionally common among workers in the aniline dye industry and this eventually led to the identification of aromatic amines as carcinogens.

The association of irradiations with cancer began to be suspected in the early years of the century. Many cases of skin cancer occurred in medical personnel who sometimes operated under x-rays. A notorious incident was an outbreak of cancer among women involved in painting watch dials with a preparation of luminous paint containing radium and thorium. It was common practice among these women to point the brushes with their tongue and a high proportion of them eventually died of a variety of tumours with a particularly high incidence of osteogenic sarcomas.

GEOGRAPHICAL DISTRIBUTION

There are considerable variations in deaths from cancer throughout the world (table 3.2) and marked differences in the incidence of many common cancers (table 3.3). A few cancers exhibit a very striking geographical distribution. One of the most remarkable is Burkitt's lymphoma. This tumour is almost entirely confined to young Africans living in the highlands of Kenya and Uganda. The tumours affect lymph glands, usually in the neck, which become infiltrated with lymphoma cells and become grossly enlarged. This tumour

Table 3.2　Deaths from cancer in various countries throughout the world. Age adjusted death rates per 100 000 population. (American Cancer Society)

Country	Males	Females
Scotland	202.8	124.6
England	182.5	114.9
USA	150.6	106.7
Australia	143.2	96.9
Japan	141.3	94.9
Norway	124.7	100.1
Portugal	113.6	84.0
Mexico	53.8	71.9

provides a very good illustration of the problems of identifying a causative factor because several factors have been correlated with it; any or all, or none, of them may be implicated in the causation of the disease. First, as Burkitt pointed out, the incidence of the lymphoma is correlated with the incidence of chronic malarial splenomegaly and he has postulated that this may be, in some way, related to the disease. Also, individuals with Burkitt's lymphoma have invariably been infected with a virus, called the Epstein–Barr virus after its discoverers. However, this virus is very widespread and has been identified as the causative agent of infectious mononucleosis, itself a proliferative disease of haemopoietic cells. Seventy per cent of adults in the United States and Northwestern Europe have antibodies to the virus and have obviously been infected at some time yet Burkitt's lymphoma is virtually unknown in these regions. The relationship between the virus and the disease is, therefore, unclear and some workers have even suggested that an entirely

Table 3.3　Incidence of common cancers in various countries. Age adjusted death rate per 100 000 population. (American Cancer Society)

Countries	Breast	Stomach (male)	Colon (male)	Lung (male)
Scotland	22.80	25.9	24.77	78.14
England	24.58	22.7	21.36	69.66
USA	21.83	9.5	18.79	40.24
Australia	19.15	15.4	18.18	37.64
Japan	3.99	65.4	8.22	13.97
Norway	16.78	25.2	13.47	14.93
Portugal	11.93	32.2	11.80	10.91
Mexico	4.18	10.1	2.76	7.30

different virus may be the cause. The favoured hypothesis (although it is by no means certain that it is correct) is that the Epstein–Barr virus is the causative agent but that, in people with a normal immune response, the cellular transformation characteristic of Burkitt's lymphoma does not occur. However, the immunosuppression which accompanies chronic malarial splenomegaly permits transformed cells to survive and become established as a tumour. The geographical distribution of Burkitt's lymphoma has provided a useful clue about the cause of the disease but the conflicting ideas being entertained indicate the problems of identifying the cause after the existence of one has been established.

Hepatomas provide another interesting example of geographical distribution. This tumour of the liver is extremely rare in most countries but is quite common in some parts of Africa. It is correlated with two factors, a generally low level of nutrition and the consumption of stored ground nuts. Some years ago it was discovered that some stored ground nuts, when fed to turkeys, produced an acute disease which was traced to a toxin produced by a fungus with which they were infected. The toxin, aflatoxin, was later shown to be able to cause hepatomas in rats and in rainbow trout in which the correlation between hepatoma and ground nut feeding had previously been observed. Therefore, it is thought that it is probably the cause of hepatoma in areas where the incidence is high and ground nuts are used as food.

Yet another example of geographical variation in incidence is provided by squamous epithelioma, a cancer of the skin, which is very much commoner in sunny tropical climates than in more northern or less sunny areas. It is also much commoner in whites than in people with darker skins. The carcinogenic factor is ultraviolet radiation but there is obviously a genetic element too. Indeed, in one particular condition, xeroderma pigmentosum, which will be referred to in a later chapter, there is a particularly high incidence of skin cancer which is greatly aggravated by exposure to the sun's rays. This provides a good example of the way in which two factors, one environmental and one genetic, may interact.

CLUSTERING IN TIME

The incidence of cancer does not remain constant. Figure 3.1(a) and (b) shows clearly how, during this century, cancer of the stomach in both sexes has progressively declined in the United States as has cancer of the uterus in women. In contrast, cancer of the lung has increased enormously during the same period in men.

Perhaps the most widely known example of clustering in time and place was the occurrence of leukaemia in survivors of the atom bombs in Hiroshima and Nagasaki. The correlation of these cases with the event leaves no room for doubt that the cause of the leukaemia in this case was radiation from the bombs.

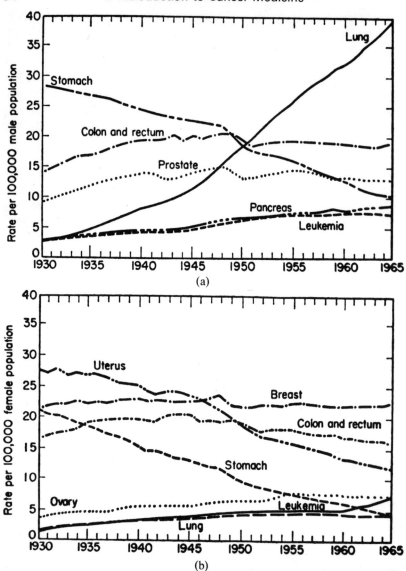

Figure 3.1   Comparison of cancer death rates by site in (a) males and (b) females in USA between the years 1930 and 1965. (*J. Am. Med. Assoc.*, **203,** 34, 1968)

Another kind of time correlation is seen in the incidence of cancer at different ages. Some kinds of cancer, such as neuroblastoma, occur almost entirely in children but the majority of cancers increase cumulatively with age. Although the reason for this is not certain, it seems very likely that it is due to the accumulation of exposure to carcinogenic factors. This is well exemplified by the incidence of cancer of the lung which is almost directly related to the number of cigarettes smoked. Hence, it is related both to the smoking habits of the individual and to his age. In general, the incidence and mortality from cancer rise steeply with age except for a small peak during the first five years of life.

OCCUPATIONAL CANCER

The earliest important correlation of this kind on record was the observation by Percival Pott, referred to earlier. Since the original observation, very many

Table 3.4   Occupations carrying an increased risk of developing cancer by site

Site	Agent	Occupation
Liver	Arsenic	Tanners, smelters
	Vinyl chloride	Plastics workers
Nasal cavity and sinuses	Chromium	Glass, pottery
	Nickel	Battery makers, electrolysis workers
	Wood and leather dust	Wood, leather, shoe workers
Lung	Arsenic, asbestos, chromium, coal dust, mustard gas, nickel, ionising radiations	Miners, asbestos workers, glass and pottery workers, coal tar and pitch workers, iron foundry, radiologists, chemical workers
Bladder	Coal products	Asphalt, coal tar
	Aromatic amines	Dyestuff users, rubber workers, leather and shoe makers, paint manufacturers
Bone	Ionising radiations	Radium dial painters
Bone marrow	Benzene, ionising radiations	Benzene workers, dye users, painters, radiologists
Skin	Coal tar, ultraviolet rays, arsenic, ionising radiations	Stokers, pitch workers, miners, outdoor workers, radiologists

occupational causes of cancer have been identified. Another particularly well-known example mentioned earlier is that of the miners in Schneeberg whose high incidence of cancer of the lung was related to high levels of radioactive uranium isotopes in dust.

Many industrial hazards are now recognised. Some occupations with an increased cancer risk are listed in table 3.4. Many of these are now carefully regulated by industrial legislation.

RACE AND ENVIRONMENT

Chronic lymphatic leukaemia is rare in Japan compared with the United States. The incidence of cancer of the colon is also much lower in Japan but the incidence of gastric cancer is higher. Are these differences in incidence due to inherited differences in susceptibility to cancer or are they due to differences in the environment? This kind of question is sometimes quite difficult to answer because, in most countries, there is a relatively genetically homogeneous majority group with similar habits and customs, exposed to much the same climatic conditions and other general environmental influences. However, a comparison of incidence of disease among emigrants with people in their country of origin can sometimes be very revealing. Chronic lymphatic leukaemia is not only rare among native Japanese but is also rare among Japanese-Americans. Hence, in this instance, it seems quite likely that some inherited factor is involved. On the other hand, second or third generation Japanese-Americans have the same high incidence of carcinoma of the colon as other Americans and this disease would, therefore, seem to be related to some factor in the environment. Indeed, there is a very good correlation between the incidence of cancer of the colon and eating habits in the more prosperous Western countries where low roughage diets are common in contrast to the high roughage diets which are common in Japan.

SEX DIFFERENCES

The common occurrence of cancers of the sex organs, such as carcinoma of the breast and carcinoma of the prostate, might be expected to affect the overall incidence but, on average, cancer occurs with equal frequency in both sexes. Men have a higher mortality rate, mainly because they have a higher incidence of cancers with poor survival rates (e.g. lung and gastrointestinal tracts). The incidence varies in the two sexes with age, being higher in males below the age of 10, higher in women between 20 and 60 and much higher in men over 60.

Marriage and child-bearing affect the incidence of some tumours as discussed below.

SOCIAL CUSTOMS

As mentioned earlier, the high incidence of mammary cancer in nuns was noted over two hundred year ago. This observation has been extended to a general negative correlation between early child-bearing and cancer of the breast. More recently, Weinberg in Stuttgart, observed that cancer of the cervix was commoner in working class women. More recently still it has been shown that this correlation is with women who have had early sexual experience and many sexual partners or have been married to promiscuous husbands. This has led to the suspicion that a virus, possibly herpes simplex 2, which causes herpes genitalis, may be involved in the causation of the disease.

One of the most important correlations between social customs and incidence of cancer has, of course, been the establishment of the causal relationship between tobacco smoking and cancer of the lung. Recognition of the relationship between the use of tobacco and the incidence of certain cancers is by no means new. Cancer of the nose in snuff users was described in the 18th century and pipe smoking was recognised to be the cause of cancer of the lower lip towards the end of that century. However, the statistical correlation between lung cancer and smoking was not demonstrated until about 1940. The studies by Doll and Hill in Great Britain and Lever, Goldstein and Gerhart, and Wynder and Graham in the United States have established this relationship between cigarette smoking and cancer of the lung beyond all reasonable doubt. Indeed, the presence of chemical carcinogens in tobacco smoke has been clearly demonstrated.

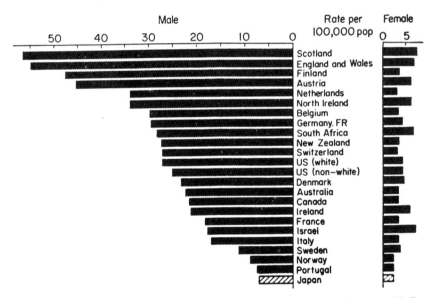

Figure 3.2   Lung cancer death rates (1956–57) in various countries (Hueper, W. C., *Occupational and Environmental Cancers of the Respiratory System*, Recent Results in Cancer Research, vol. 3, Springer–Verlag, Heidelberg, 1966)

Cancer of the lung provides an illustration of many epidemiological phenomena. The incidence in different countries varies enormously (figure 3.2). The remarkable increase in cancer of the lung during this century in the USA, illustrated in figure 3.1, has already been alluded to. Another facet of

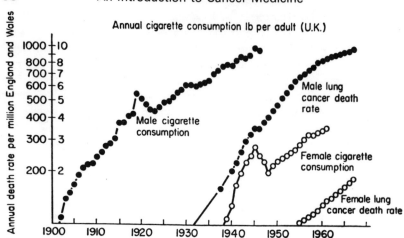

Figure 3.3 Comparison of the annual death rate from lung cancer in males and females with the rate of consumption of tobacco. (HMSO, London, 1968)

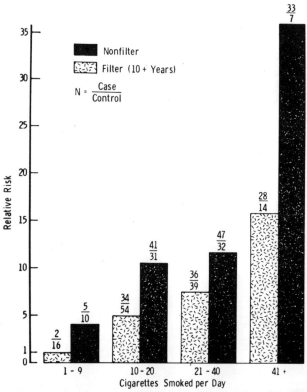

Figure 3.4 Relative risk of lung cancer among current smokers in relation to the number of cigarettes smoked per day (males 1966–71). (Wynder, E. L., Mabuchi, K. and Hoffman, D., in *Cancer Epidemiology and Protection* (Ed. D. Schottenfeld), Thomas, Springfield, Illinois, 1975, p. 121)

this, shown in figure 3.3, is that in Britain the rise in lung cancer among men followed about thirty years behind a similar increase in consumption of cigarettes. This also shows the beginning of a similar trend in women, following about fifteen years behind a dramatic increase in consumption of cigarettes among women which started at the beginning of World War II. The relationship has now been clearly established by 'prospective' studies. In these, the smoking habits of large groups were recorded and then as these people died, the cause of death was related to smoking habits. These studies very clearly demonstrated the greatly increased risk of cancer of the lung incurred by habitual smokers and, indeed, showed a close correlation between the death rate from this cause and the number of cigarettes smoked (figure 3.4).

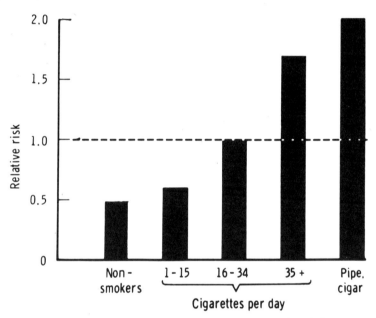

Figure 3.5   Relative risk of developing cancer of the mouth in relation to smoking habits. (Wynder, E. L., Bross, I. J. and Feldman, R. M., *Cancer*, **10**, 1300, 1957)

Cancer of the lung is only the most striking of a number of diseases associated with smoking. Cancer of the mouth exhibits a similar relationship as is clearly shown in figure 3.5.

4 Physical and Chemical Causes

RADIATIONS

Ever since Friebin in 1902 reported the occurrence of an epidermoid carcinoma on the hand of a radiologist, it has been appreciated that certain radiations can cause cancers. In the early days of x-rays, radiologists often adjusted their equipment with their hands exposed to the beam. Surgeons even operated for foreign bodies under the x-ray machine. As a result, within fifteen years of Röntgen's discovery (by 1911) over 90 cases of skin cancer in radiologists, surgeons and radiation technicians had been reported. Most of these were squamous carcinomas and basal cell carcinomas but there were also some fibrosarcomas. Subsequently, other episodes reinforced this evidence that x-rays cause cancer. Some have already been discussed in chapter 3, including the occurrence of cancer of the lung in miners working with radioactive ores, of osteosarcomas in women painting clock faces with a radioactive paint and, of course, the aftermath of the atomic bombs. The clinical observations in humans have been reinforced by experimental observations in cultured cells and in animals, from which it appears that radiations can produce almost any kind of tumour.

There are two general kinds of radiation, electromagnetic radiations and corpuscular or particulate radiations. Electromagnetic radiations include ultraviolet, visible and infrared light, radio waves, x-rays and microwaves. Of these, only ultraviolet light and so-called ionising radiations (gamma rays and x-rays) appear to be carcinogenic. Ultraviolet light at a wavelength of about two hundred and sixty nanometres is strongly absorbed by nucleic acids and the major effect of ultraviolet light is on them. One of the commonest reactions is the formation of covalent bonds between pairs of pyrimidines (thymine, cytosine and uracil).

Ionising radiations carry energy sufficient to enable them to displace electrons from atoms, thus converting them to ions. (Since electrons carry a negative charge when they are removed from neutral atoms, this means that the remaining particles are also charged. These are ions and they are chemically highly reactive.) They can catalyse very many radiochemical reactions and probably interact with nearly all molecules in the cell in a random way. Since most proteins and RNA molecules are present in thousands of copies in the cell, random damage to them is not particularly serious unless extremely high doses of irradiation are given because many undamaged molecules remain. With DNA, however, it is another matter. Ionisation can give rise to many different chemical changes in DNA, resulting in changes in bases, cross-linking between DNA strands and degradation. Since most genes are present as only two copies in each cell and sometimes as only one, damage to DNA can have very serious effects; this is probably how most of the obvious damage by ionising radiations is caused.

Corpuscular radiation is formed by the emission from atoms of particles such as α-particles, β-particles, protons and neutrons. These particles carry a large amount of energy with them but, apart from this and the fact that they are less penetrating, the effects are generally much the same as those of ionising electromagnetic radiation. Different radiations have different relative effects. They can be characterised by their 'linear energy transfer' or LET. The LET is related to the relative biological efficiency (RBE) of radiations in that the more densely ionising radiations, i.e. those with the higher values for LET, also have a higher relative biological efficiency, that is, they produce tumours with higher efficiency.

The damage done by radiations can result in cell death and this is the basis of radiotherapy. Cancerous changes are produced by much lower doses which damage only a very few cells in such a way that, while they can survive, they are permanently altered. Both in radiotherapy and in radiation carcinogenesis, many factors influence the effectiveness of radiation. One of the most important is the rate of dosage. Generally speaking, a dose of radiation given over a very short time is much more effective than the same dose given over a much longer time. For example, in experimental animals, the time of appearance of tumours varies inversely with the dose and, moreover, the lower the rate at which the dose is given, the lower is the incidence of tumours and the longer the delay in their appearance. The reason for this is the existence in cells of mechanisms for the repair of radiation damage. These mechanisms are essential for survival because all living forms are continuously being exposed to low levels of irradiation from natural sources. They can probably cope with damage occurring at a low rate but are overwhelmed when this is too high.

Three kinds of DNA repair mechanisms have been recognised. The first is called 'enzyme catalysed photoreactivation'. This kind of repair occurs in non-dividing cells and is activated by visible light. It involves enzymes which replace damaged bases in nucleic acids.

The second kind of repair (figure 4.1) which has been very extensively studied, is called excision-repair or, commonly, 'cut and patch' repair. A specialised enzyme first recognises the presence of abnormal bases and cuts the damaged strand of DNA at that point. Another enzyme then excises the damaged sequences and some adjacent ones from that strand of DNA. Yet another enzyme replaces the bases which have been removed by synthesising a new base-paired strand complementary to the normal one. A final enzyme joins the repaired region to the adjacent undamaged DNA. A chain with so many links is vulnerable. Mutations might affect any component and the condition xeroderma pigmentosum, mentioned in chapter 3 and described more fully in chapter 6, is due to hereditary absence of one or other of these enzymes.

The third kind of repair is 'replication' repair. The details of this process are not known but it appears that, in this instance, the DNA is repaired as it is being replicated prior to cell division.

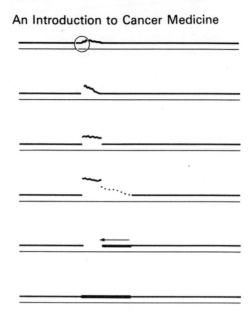

Figure 4.1   'Cut and patch' repair of DNA

Exposure to radiation, such as to give rise to cancer, occurs in a variety of circumstances. Occupational cancer among the early radiologists has already been referred to. Because of this experience, very stringent safeguards are now enforced to reduce or prevent exposure among radiologists, radiotherapists, people working with radioactive isotopes and workers in processes which involve a risk of exposure to radiation. Nevertheless, accidental exposure does sometimes occur in these occupations (for example, as a result of leaks in atomic plants). Another notorious example of accidental exposure occurred in the Marshal Islands where a large number of natives were exposed to fall-out from an atomic explosion. This included a large proportion of radioactive iodine and many of them developed thyroid cancers, since iodine is concentrated in the thyroid gland.

The commonest form of exposure in most countries today comes from therapeutic and diagnostic x-rays. An increased incidence of leukaemia has been well documented in patients receiving radiotherapy for ankylosing spondylitis and it has been shown that children exposed *in utero* to x-rays have a significant (though barely detectable) increase in incidence of a variety of tumours. The greatest potential risk is, of course, wartime exposure. One atomic or hydrogen bomb can expose a population to far more irradiation damage than the whole population of the world is likely to experience from all other causes.

The carcinogenic effects of irradiations have been thoroughly documented and quantified over the past twenty or thirty years but they are by no means the only physical factors which can cause cancer. Since the beginning of the century it has been recognised that cancers can arise in relation to foreign bodies, scars and chronic inflammation. Besides these observations in man, extensive experimental studies have been undertaken on the implantation of inert plastics into rodents and it has been shown that these regularly give rise to sarcomas. The precise mechanism whereby most of these factors cause cancer is not understood. It is probably quite different from those described above and may, for example, have to do with some interference with the intercellular signals which are necessary for normal tissue differentiation.

CHEMICAL CARCINOGENS

In chapter 3 epidemiological evidence was discussed which implicates tars, oils and a variety of other substances in the production of cancer. Since the beginning of this century, a great deal of work has gone into identifying the active chemicals in these substances. It was originally hoped that a few substances with common features would be identified as carcinogens. However, a very large number of cancer-inducing chemicals have been discovered (see table 3.4) and it is very difficult indeed to see what these substances have in common. In fact, it is only very recently that a rational explanation for the diversity of chemical carcinogens has emerged. An important event in improving our understanding was the discovery that carcinogens can be divided into those which act directly on tissue constituents and those which are not themselves directly effective but are altered by metabolic processes to give rise to effective carcinogens. The former, described as direct-acting carcinogens are, without exception, highly reactive chemicals. They include carcinogens such as β-propiolactone, dimethylsulphate and nitrogen mustard, all of which can react directly with nucleic acids and proteins. Chemically, all the substances in this group are described as electrophilic, which means that they readily participate in reactions in which they take up electrons. As will be described later, this property not only enables them to react very widely with many chemicals but especially to interact in a fairly specific way with nucleic acids.

The second group of carcinogens, which need to be chemically modified before they become active, are described as procarcinogens. This implies that they have to be metabolically converted to active forms, which are called 'ultimate' carcinogens. Commonly, intermediate compounds called 'proximate' carcinogens are formed (figure 4.2). Many of the substances ingested from plants and vegetables would be highly toxic if not rapidly modified in the body. All animals have therefore developed mechanisms for dealing with the many foreign and sometimes harmful chemicals they encounter in their natural environment. There are two main kinds of these reactions. One involves an internal chemical modification of the molecule, for example, by oxidation, reduction, hydroxylation or degradation. Many of these reactions occur in the liver in which a special machinery associated with the microsomes is responsible. This machinery utilises a special molecule,

44

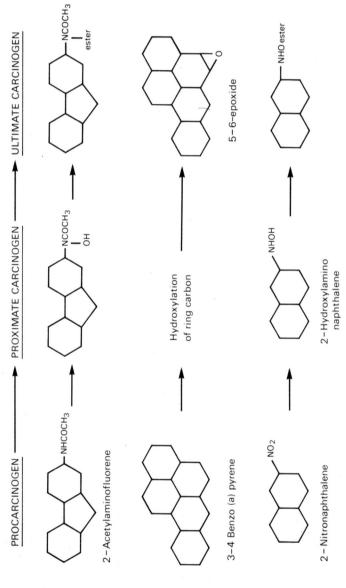

Figure 4.2   Metabolic modifications of carcinogens which give rise to highly reactive molecules

PROCARCINOGEN ⟶ PROXIMATE CARCINOGEN ⟶ ULTIMATE CARCINOGEN

NHCOCH₃

2 – Acetylaminofluorene

NCOCH₃
OH

NCOCH₃
ester

3 – 4 Benzo (a) pyrene

Hydroxylation
of ring carbon

O

5–6-epoxide

NO₂

2 – Nitronaphthalene

NHOH

2 – Hydroxylamino
naphthalene

NHO ester

cytochrome P450, and is referred to as the cytochrome P450 system. It is particularly involved in oxidation and hydroxylation reactions.

The other major detoxication process is conjugation; it involves linking toxic molecules to other molecules, such as acetic, sulphuric or glucuronic acid to form acetate, sulphate or glucuronide esters. These conjugates are often highly soluble, less toxic than the original products and easily excreted. These detoxication systems were evolved over many millions of years to deal with natural products in the environment and render them harmless but the environment of our present technological world contains high concentrations of new kinds of chemicals. Many of these are modified biochemically by the body by enzymes evolved to deal with substances which occur naturally but this modification is not now necessarily harmless. Indeed, some of the products of tars and oils, when modified by these systems, are more harmful than the parent compounds. For example, substances of the kind called heterocyclic hydrocarbons include chemicals like benzo-anthracene. Benzo-anthracene itself is not a very active carcinogen, but it is converted by the mechanisms described above to an oxidised derivative (an epoxide) which is highly chemically active and is the ultimate carcinogen (figure 4.2). Many other procarcinogens are first hydroxylated and then converted to esters (with sulphate or glucuronic acid) which are the active compounds. The ultimate carcinogens, like the direct-acting carcinogens, are electrophilic substances. The groups with which they react are called 'nucleophilic'. These are groups which readily combine with electrophilic reagents and give up electrons to them. Nucleophilic groups occur in proteins and nucleic acids. Many ultimate carcinogens react particularly readily with the four bases of DNA, notably with one particular nitrogen atom in guanine (figure 4.3). As a result of these reactions, most of these compounds form strong chemical bonds (covalent bonds) with the DNA bases. For example, the substance dimethylnitrosamine is a particularly potent carcinogen. It undergoes rapid changes in tissue to yield an active methyl group, called a methyl-carbonium ion which reacts with guanine to form 7-methyl-guanine. These modifications of bases in DNA affect the properties of the DNA and therefore have far-reaching effects on the cell in the same way as ionising radiation.

Not all chemical carcinogens react with DNA in exactly the same way and there is another group which produces its effect by sliding between bases in the Watson–Crick DNA structure. This is called intercalation; it has the effect of disturbing the structure and therefore the behaviour of DNA.

The discovery that nearly all chemical carcinogens can give rise to highly active substances which interact with nucleic acids and proteins suggests a common mode of action. It was previously almost impossible to explain why metals like nickel and chromium, as well as complicated organic substances like methylcholanthrene, are carcinogenic. However, some of these metals behave as electrophilic substances towards nucleic acids while methylcholanthrene probably intercalates with DNA. It is now fairly certain, therefore, that all direct-acting and ultimate carcinogens produce their effects

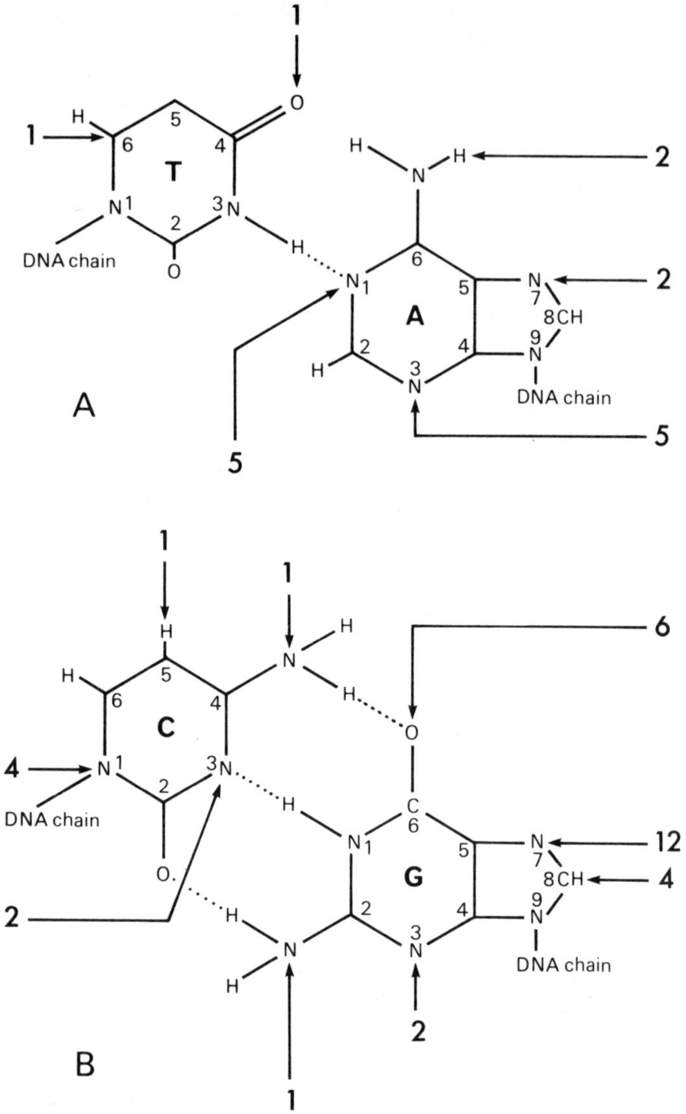

Figure 4.3 Sites of reactivity with carcinogens in purine nucleotides. The numbers indicate the number of modifications caused by carcinogenic chemicals at the position.

by altering DNA, that is, they are mutagens. However, it should not be thought that this hypothesis has been proven. Although a very likely explanation for the mode of action of very many carcinogens, it is by no means the only one possible.

One of the puzzling things about carcinogens has been the fact that individual chemicals often produce tumours in specific sites in the body which are sometimes far distant from the route of administration. Now that we have more knowledge of the comparative biochemical pharmacology of these compounds, we can see explanations. The detoxication pathways which have been referred to are mainly present in the kidney and liver, predominantly in the latter. This is probably why so many carcinogens, however administered, produce tumours in the liver in experimental animals. After the substances have been modified and conjugated as esters, they are then excreted either in the bile or in the urine and the extent to which they are secreted by either route is very often a function of the species of animal. Dimethylaminobiphenyl produces mainly intestinal cancers in rats but urinary cancers in hamsters. This almost certainly reflects a predominantly biliary excretion in rats and a predominantly urinary excretion in hamsters. The size of the molecules also influences the route of excretion. Larger molecules pass out in the bile; for example, more dichlorobenzidine than benzidine is found in the bile of dogs whereas more benzidine is excreted in the urine. Hence, the different ways of processing different compounds probably explain, in large measure, why they produce lesions in different parts of the body.

Individual susceptibility to carcinogens may also be determined by the capacity to modify them. An interesting example relates to the enzyme aryl hydrocarbon hydroxylase. This enzyme increases in amount (i.e. is induced) in cells from most people when treated with certain inducers. However, some people have an inherited defect which is exhibited by a failure of induction. There is evidence that these individuals are less susceptible to the carcinogens in tobacco smoke.

The action of bacteria in modifying chemicals in the gut is probably of very great importance. Some substances, inactivated by being conjugated as esters, are excreted in the bile; they are then rapidly broken down by bacteria in the gut to yield active compounds again. In a similar way, non-toxic substances ingested in the food may sometimes be converted to toxic ones by bacteria. For example, nitrates used as preservatives in food may be used by bacteria to form the highly carcinogenic nitroso compounds.

The evidence very strongly points to most ultimate chemical carcinogens being mutagens and this hypothesis has stimulated attempts to exploit genetic systems to recognise potentially carcinogenic substances. Because most carcinogens have to be biochemically altered to reveal their potential mutagenicity, the first step in these assays is incubation of the possible carcinogen with a biochemical preparation from liver containing the metabolic enzymes which carry out the modifications. The mixture, now expected to contain the ultimate carcinogen, is then tested on a suitable system, such as tissue culture cells, to determine whether transformation is caused. The Ames assay, which has been developed along these lines, does not use mammalian cells at all but relies on the use of special 'marker' bacteria which are very sensitive to mutagens and show an easily detected change in their presence. By use of assays of this kind, evidence has been obtained quite recently that a number of commonly available commercial items, such as hair dyes, may contain quite potent pro-carcinogens.

Although evidence is accumulating that most chemical carcinogens can act as mutagens, the opposite is not necessarily true. For example, hydroxylamine is a powerful mutagen in bacteria but is not carcinogenic, possibly because in animal cells it is very rapidly bound to proteins in the cell.

COCARCINOGENS

A few carcinogens are so powerful that a single brief exposure is enough to ensure the development of tumours in experimental animals, but most require repeated exposure. Moreover, in some cases, a combination of two carcinogens is much more effective than would be expected simply by adding together the individual effects of each. Even more puzzling, some substances which are not carcinogenic at all by themselves have the property of greatly potentiating the action of known carcinogens. These are called cocarcinogens. They are effective if administered simultaneously with carcinogens but what is even more puzzling is that cocarcinogens will produce their effects if administered some time after carcinogens. One of the best known substances to behave in this way is croton oil which itself is not carcinogenic. If mice are given a single treatment with a carcinogen on the skin, then cancer may either not develop or it may arise only after a very long time interval. However, if croton oil is painted on the skin some time after the carcinogen has been administered, then a cancer develops very quickly. The carcinogen in these skin painting experiments is called the initiating factor and the croton oil the promoting factor. The promotion effect of croton oil is due to a substance which has been chemically purified (a fatty acid ester of an unusual heterocyclic hydrocarbon called phorbol).

The relationship between the initiation and promotion effects in carcinogenesis is not properly understood but it may well be very important. There is evidence that cigarette smoke contains substances with a strong promoting effect. Since this important but well-documented phenomenon is not fully understood, we have to be cautious about accepting mechanisms described earlier in this chapter as providing a full and complete explanation for physical and chemical carcinogenesis.

IATROGENIC CANCERS

'Iatrogenic' diseases are those which arise from measures used in medical treatment itself. The carcinogenic effect of radiation has already been discussed earlier in this chapter. The advantages of using radiation to cure an established cancer very greatly outweigh the slight risk of inducing cancer in a middle-aged or elderly person. However, the wanton exposure of young children to high doses of radiation is indefensible because the risk is not insignificant. As in so many things in medicine a balanced judgment of advan-

Table 4.1   Drugs related to the development of cancer in man

Drug	Related cancer
Radioisotopes	
Radium, ^{32}P	Leukaemia
Thorotrast	Osteosarcoma
Immunosuppressive drugs for renal	Reticulum cell sarcoma
transplantation etc.	Brain neoplasma etc.
Cytotoxic drugs used in cancer chemotherapy	Various
Hormones	
Oestrogens pre-natal	Vaginal and cervical adenocarcinomas
Post-natal oestrogens	Endometrial carcinoma
Androgenic anabolic steroids	Hepatocellular carcinoma
Contraceptive pill	Haemangiosarcomas of liver
Arsenic	Skin cancer
Phenacetin containing drugs	Renal cancer
Reserpine?	Breast cancer
Chloramphenicol?	Leukaemia

tages and risks has to be made, based on knowledge and experience. Besides radiation a causal connection between some therapeutic agents and cancers has either been shown or suspected and table 4.1 provides a list of these.

5 Tumour Viruses

That cancer could be caused by viruses was discovered by Ellerman and Bang in 1908 when they showed that an avian leukaemia could be transmitted by cell-free extracts. During the past twenty years, the part played by viruses in the production of cancer has been the subject of intensive research and we now know a great deal about it. Several types of virus have been implicated. They are generally divided into the DNA viruses and the RNA viruses and then subdivided within these groups. All the tumour viruses have a rather simple structure in which the nucleic acid forms an internal core or nucleoid. This is surrounded by proteins which form a viral coat or envelope called the capsid. In most tumour viruses, it has a precise geometrical structure composed of protein sub-units called capsomeres. In some viruses the whole is encased in a lipoprotein envelope. The entire viral particle is sometimes referred to as a virion (figure 5.1).

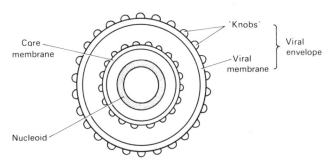

Figure 5.1   Schematic diagram of a tumour virus

DNA tumour viruses are conveniently separated into two groups, the small viruses called the papova viruses which contain about three million daltons of DNA and the large ones which contain about four times as much. The former include the papilloma viruses (which cause warts) and the polyoma and SV40 viruses (important in experimental cancer research); the latter include the adenoviruses and the herpes type viruses associated with Burkitt's lymphoma of humans and Marek's disease of chickens.

SMALL DNA VIRUSES (PAPOVA VIRUSES)

A very great deal of our present knowledge of viral carcinogenesis derives from studies of polyoma and SV40 viruses. Polyoma virus occurs spontaneously in mice and, as its name implies, it causes a wide range of tumours in them. Mice which are infected with polyoma virus do not always develop tumours but excrete live polyoma virus in the urine. Hence, many mouse stocks are chronically infected with it. The virus can also induce tumours in other rodents, for example, hamsters and guinea pigs if administered to them in large doses. In hamsters, it commonly causes kidney tumours but, in contrast with the mouse, after tumours have been induced, the virus apparently disappears. It is never excreted in the urine and it has not proved possible to recover it from the tumours or other tissues of affected hamsters.

One of the most important findings in tumour virus research was the observation that something akin to carcinogenesis can be reproduced in tissue cultures of baby hamster kidney cells. The phenomenon is called transformation (figure 2.11) and was described in chapter 2. These cells are fibroblastic in type. When inoculated with polyoma virus, foci develop with cells of different morphology and growth pattern. Moreover, if cells which have been transformed in this way are inoculated into the brains of baby hamsters, they readily form tumours even when only a very few cells are introduced. When transformed cells are cloned (i.e. colonies are grown from single cells), the clones generally retain the transformed morphology and behaviour indefinitely. As in the adult hamster, intact polyoma virus cannot be recovered from transformed baby hamster kidney cells. However, if a similar experiment is done with mouse fibroblasts, lytic foci form from which polyoma virions are released. Hence, the difference in behaviour between the mouse and hamster is reflected in a difference in behaviour of their isolated cells. Apparently the hamster lacks some mechanism which is present in the mouse and which is necessary for the virus to complete its normal replicative cycle. The abortive cycle nevertheless results in the expression of some viral functions and gives rise to the phenomenon of transformation which, in many respects, resembles natural carcinogenesis.

What happens to the DNA from the tumour virus in transformed cells? The answer to this has been found by using a technique called nucleic acid hybridisation. This is a method in which one nucleic acid is matched with another in much the same way as a photocopy of a page of a book can be matched with the page itself. It depends on the relationship, described in chapter 2, between one strand and another of DNA, or between DNA and the RNA formed from it, that is guanine always base-pairs with cytosine and adenine always base-pairs with thymine or uracil. It is a technique which can be used to search for a known nucleic acid and it has much the same specificity as exists between a photocopy and the page from which it was taken. When it is used to search for the polyoma viral DNA in transformed cells, it is found that while no viral nucleic acid can be found free in the cytoplasm or in the nuclear sap, it can nevertheless be found in the DNA of the host cell itself. Apparently, the viral DNA has in some way been stitched into the genome so as to form an integral part of it. In fact, transformed cells contain several copies of polyoma virus DNA in the genome, a phenomenon which has a very close parallel in bacteria. Some bacterial viruses can grow free within the cell in one set of circumstances and in another can become integrated into the bacterial DNA. In certain special conditions, the process can then be reversed; the viral DNA can be cut out from the bacterial DNA to reproduce again in the free form and cause lysis of the bacterium. Although this process of excision has not been observed with the polyoma virus, it has been demonstrated with SV40.

The SV40 virus is very similar to the polyoma virus and of about the same size. It is a simian virus and was discovered in tissue cultures of monkey kidney which were being used to prepare the Salk poliomyelitis vaccine. Fortunately, no evidence has emerged that this virus gives rise to tumours in human beings although many thousands of people receiving the Salk vaccine were inadvertently infected with it and this group has been under close scrutiny for many years. In tissue cultures of human or baby hamster fibroblasts, SV40 virus produces transformation which, in nearly all respects, seems to be identical to the transformation produced by polyoma virus in baby hamster kidney cells. Following transformation it is not possible to demonstrate free virus in the hamster cells although, as with the polyoma virus, copies of it can be found in the genome of these cells. However, in certain other cells, notably cells derived from green monkeys, SV40 can give rise to a productive infection, i.e. free infectious virus is produced. This has made it possible to perform an experiment which demonstrates that the SV40 virus can be rescued from the genome of the hamster cell. In this experiment, untransformed monkey kidney cells were fused to hamster cells transformed with SV40 virus so as to give rise to a monkey/hamster hybrid cell. Although free virus could not be demonstrated in the hamster parent, it was released from the hybrid and therefore must have been derived from it.

Both polyoma virus and SV40 virus are so small that it is unlikely that they contain more than seven or eight genes.

The genetics of SV40 have been extensively studied and seven functions have been demonstrated. Four of these involve information for coat proteins and are probably not important in the transformation event. Of the three others, one seems to be responsible for initiating many of the changes involved in viral transformation, a second seems to be responsible for the induction of a special antigen, the tumour-specific transplantation antigen (TSTA), and the third for another antigen which is viral and called the T-antigen. From this and similar evidence obtained from polyoma virus, it seems very likely that the transformation process depends on only one or two genes.

The papilloma viruses are the causative agents of some benign skin tumours, the best known of which is the common wart in humans.

LARGE DNA VIRUSES

The large DNA viruses which have been implicated in tumour production are mostly of the herpes type, i.e. they are similar to the virus which causes herpes simplex. The herpes viruses have about four times as much DNA as the small DNA viruses.

There has been very great interest in recent years in the role of a herpes type virus (the Epstein–Barr virus, EBV) in Burkitt's lymphoma (chapter 3). This typical herpes virus has been identified as the agent of infectious mononucleosis but it is not yet clear how this disease is related to Burkitt's lymphoma. In Burkitt's lymphoma, virtually 100 per cent of the patients have antibodies to EBV but this, by itself, is not a compelling reason to consider that the virus has anything to do with the disease as 70 per cent of adults in western countries also possess these antibodies.

An important piece of evidence for the involvement of herpes viruses in the production of cancer-like conditions comes from an epidemic disease of fowls called Marek's disease. Clinically Marek's disease involves massive lymphocytic proliferation and infiltration. One of the principal clinical consequences is paralysis due to infiltration of nerve tissue but the other major feature which interests oncologists is that the haematological picture is one of leukaemia. The disease is infectious and of great importance in the poultry industry. The agent has been positively identified as a herpes virus and it is of great importance and interest that in this disease an effective attenuated viral vaccine has been prepared which protects birds against the disease.

There have been conjectural associations of other herpes-type viruses with certain tumours. In particular it has been suggested that a form of the human herpes simplex virus (herpes simplex virus 2) may be involved in the causation of cancer of the cervix in women. However, this association is by no means certain.

The adenoviruses are of particular interest in three respects. First, many occur normally in the human where they are commonly associated with acute upper respiratory infections. Secondly, in baby hamster kidney cells and some other cells, they cause transformation very similar to that produced by polyoma or SV40 virus. Thirdly, they are themselves quite large viruses and can combine with other viruses to form hybrid viruses.

RNA TUMOUR VIRUSES (ONCORNA VIRUSES)

Two main types of RNA tumour viruses are recognised, based on slight differences in morphology. These are the B-type viruses, the typical example of which is the mouse mammary tumour virus (MMTV) and the C-type viruses, which commonly give rise to leukaemias and sarcomas in animals. (There are also A-type virus particles which are probably intracytoplasmic precursors of B-type viruses.)

The mouse mammary tumour virus was originally known as the Bittner factor. Evidence for its presence arose from observations in certain strains of mice which exhibit a very high incidence of mammary tumours. It was found that infant mice obtained by Caesarian section could be protected from the disease by suckling them with foster mothers of a resistant strain. From this observation, evidence accumulated that the disease was due to a virus transmitted to young mice in their mother's milk.

The C-type viruses include avian and murine sarcoma and leukaemia viruses. The first of this group to be described was an avian sarcoma virus, named the Rous sarcoma virus (RSV) after its discoverer. As its name implies, this virus is responsible for the transmission of sarcomas of chickens. It is a transforming virus in that it gives rise to typical transformed colonies in cultures of chick fibroblast cells. However, these are also productive colonies in that they release the virus which has been identified as the causative agent of the disease. Studies of the Rous sarcoma virus have yielded a great deal of very interesting information concerning the relationship of tumour viruses to other viruses.

The Rous virus itself is a *defective* virus, that is, it lacks certain of the functions necessary to permit it to go through a replicative cycle and produce new infective RSV particles. This pure, defective RSV can transform chick fibroblasts but never yields productive foci. In this respect, it behaves like the polyoma virus in baby hamster kidney cells. However, if not highly purified, RSV is associated with another virus called the Rous-associated virus (RAV), which provides the functions missing in RSV and permits completion of the replicative cycle. Hence, cells treated with pure RSV show only transformation whereas cells treated with crude preparations also containing RAV or intentionally co-infected with RSV + RAV give rise to foci from which virus is produced. RAV helps RSV to complete its cycle and viruses which complement defective viruses in this way are called 'helper' viruses. Observations of this kind with this and other viruses have led to the general hypothesis that nearly all tumour viruses are defective in cells which they transform. For example, mouse cells are 'permissive' for the polyoma virus, that is, they permit a full replicative cycle and the production of new virus particles. On the other hand, hamster cells are 'non-permissive' in the sense that these cells can be transformed by the virus but they do not produce complete virus particles. Presumably, in this instance, the mouse cells provide a function necessary for viral replication which is absent from hamster cells.

It is not difficult to understand how the genetic information of DNA viruses is inherited or how they replicate in the same way as most other organisms in which DNA is the genetic material. However, the RNA viruses present a problem because they do not seem to fit into the general pattern in which the genetic material is DNA. The problem has been solved by the discovery that these viruses contain within the virion an enzyme, RNA-dependent DNA polymerase, more commonly known as reverse transcriptase, which is capable of synthesising a double-stranded DNA molecule from the viral RNA. The first event after one of these RNA viruses has entered a cell, and its coat has been removed, is the synthesis of a DNA copy. This DNA intermediate is called a pro-virus; like the DNA of DNA viruses, it can be integrated into the genome of the host. Consequently, in cells which have been transformed by RNA viruses, one can demonstrate by the nucleic acid

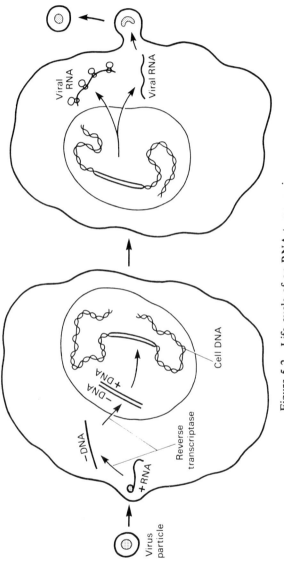

Figure 5.2   Life cycle of an RNA tumour virus

hybridisation technique that DNA sequences corresponding to the viral RNA are present in the DNA in the chromosomes in the cell nucleus (figure 5.2).

REVERSION

Although the Rous sarcoma virus normally affects chicken cells, it can also transform cells of a wide variety of other vertebrates. One strain in particular, the Schmidt–Ruppin strain, can even transform baby hamster kidney cells. It might be suspected that the virus would have only a very tenuous hold on these cells and, indeed, if the transformed cells are plated out in such a way that single cells give rise to colonies, it is found that quite a high proportion of the colonies behave like untransformed cells. This very interesting phenomenon is called reversion. It has been studied in a more systematic way be preparing temperature-sensitive mutants of the virus. These temperature-sensitive mutants possess a temperature-sensitive function which is important in transformation. When cells transformed with these viruses are grown at a 'permissive' temperature, usually a temperature lower than body temperature, they exhibit all the phenomena characteristic of transformed cells but if the temperature is raised to a 'non-permissive' temperature, at which the temperature-sensitive property does not function, then they assume the appearance of normal cells. Experiments of a similar kind have been done with DNA viruses, particularly polyoma and SV40. They indicate that the process which gives rise to transformation can be completely reversed. Moreover, they imply that transformation depends on probably only one viral function.

TRANSMISSION OF VIRUSES: THE ONCOGENE HYPOTHESIS

There is now evidence that tumour viruses can be transmitted in at least two and possibly three ways (figure 5.3). Horizontal transmission, that is, direct infection of one animal by another, most obviously occurs in Marek's disease and in polyoma infection. Marek's disease is an epidemic disease and it has already been discussed; it is not certain that it should be considered as a neoplasm. However, the polyoma virus can be transmitted horizontally in mice and, in this instance, there is no doubt that it gives rise to tumours. In the human, the Epstein–Barr virus is also transmitted horizontally but perhaps the best known human tumour which can be transmitted by direct infection is the common wart caused by the papilloma virus. All these are DNA viruses.

Among RNA viruses, fowl leukaemia viruses are almost certainly also transmitted horizontally and there is quite strong evidence that this is true of cat leukaemia. As mentioned in chapter 3 intensive studies have been pursued with a view to determining whether any of the more important human cancers are infective, notably leukaemia and Hodgkin's disease, but although one or

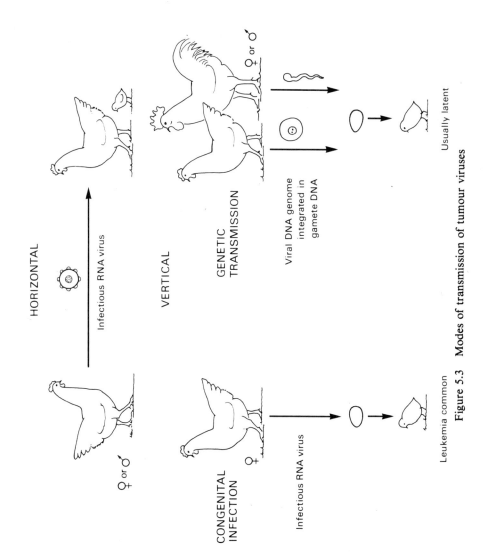

Figure 5.3 Modes of transmission of tumour viruses

two striking examples of apparent clustering have been reported, no hard and fast conclusions have been reached.

The second mode of transmission is vertical transmission which involves infection of progeny from parents. Reference has been made to this mode of transmission in mouse mammary tumours in which the virus is passed on to sucklings in the mother's milk. In a strict sense, this form of infection is not very different from horizontal infection since the infected animal receives free virus from its environment.

The avian leukosis virus can not only be transmitted horizontally, it can be transmitted to progeny through the egg and sperm (figure 5.3). Hence, in this instance, vertical infection is not analogous to horizontal transmission; moreover, there is no simple way of breaking the chain of infection. This is a truly vertical transmission.

When the nucleic acid hybridisation method was used to search for the presence of Rous sarcoma pro-virus, a surprising result was obtained. It emerged that some RSV sequences are present in the genome of all fowls tested whether they have been exposed to RSV or not. This included some which are so far removed from each other in evolution that they must have diverged hundreds of thousands or even millions of years ago.

In studies concerned with murine leukaemia and sarcoma viruses, a similar but not identical phenomenon has been discovered. When cultured mouse cells were treated in ways known to release integrated viruses, virus particles were indeed produced but these were shown not to be well-known mouse tumour viruses (although related to them). They are called endogenous viruses, and their nature is obscure, but it appears that some of these endogenous viruses have extraordinary characteristics. They are not infectious for the species from which they are derived but will infect cells of other species and will sometimes cause transformation. Viruses which behave in this way are called xenotropic viruses.

Linked to this finding is the further observation that nucleic acid sequences corresponding to clearly identified viruses in one species turn up as components of the genome in quite different species. One very remarkable example of this is that sequences corresponding to the cat leukaemia virus occur in the DNA of old-world monkeys. These observations have led to the suspicion that viruses which can cause acute infectious diseases in one species may infect an unrelated species which is non-permissive for replication and that, in these species, they may behave as transforming viruses or may become integrated into the DNA without causing transformation.

Another related phenomenon is that some viruses, for example the mouse leukaemia viruses, can cause the appearance of antigens which are characteristic of viruses of the entire group. They are called group-specific antigens, and proteins with the same characteristics can be identified in normal and infected animals in embryonic development. There is, therefore, the possibility that some of these viral sequences may be related to genetic information which is normally used.

Stimulated by these findings, much interest has centred recently on the possibility that many tumour viruses may be inherited as pro-virus-like sequences integrated into the DNA of the genome. According to the oncogene hypothesis, tumour virus RNA sequences have been integrated into the DNA of distant ancestors of the present generation and then inherited through the germ line, with the result that all present day individuals carry them. It is postulated that these virus sequences normally remain dormant but may be activated by carcinogens − either chemical carcinogens or viruses which provide the necessary functions. Although there is no direct evidence that the oncogene hypothesis is correct, there is no doubt that a situation very similar to that predicted by the hypothesis exists in fowls.

6 Genetic Factors

Cancer cells behave very much like normal cells which have undergone a mutation and become altered in an inherited fashion. Indeed, as discussed later, one of the major theories of cancer is the somatic mutation hypothesis, the implications of which are as follows. Heredity, as we normally think of it, is determined by properties of the germinal cell line. Characteristics such as eye or hair colour, while expressed in the somatic cells (the differentiated cells of the mature organism), are passed down from generation to generation through the sex cells or gametes. From the hereditary point of view, changes in the genetic material of somatic cells are unimportant because they are never inherited in the next generation. From the point of view of cancer production, however, such changes may be crucial.

It does not require very many cell divisions to form the major organs in the mature individual from a fertilised egg but in some tissues in the adult animal, such as the bone marrow, cells continue to divide at a high rate. Hence, an alteration in the genes of a somatic cell from such a tissue can have repercussions some time later if the mutated cell behaves abnormally and outgrows all the others. In this way, a somatic cell mutation in a blood cell precursor, could be seen as a reasonable candidate for the production of leukaemia. Moreover, in a tissue in which the cells normally grow very slowly, a similar change could give rise to a more rapidly growing cell. The number of cells in the human body is so large and so many of them continue to divide throughout life that it would be surprising if mutations of this kind did not arise with quite high frequency. The somatic mutation hypothesis therefore seems very reasonable. This chapter discusses the evidence for genetic changes in cancer cells and for inherited predisposition to the disease.

CHROMOSOMAL CHANGES IN CANCER CELLS

The normal human karyotype (chromosome pattern) is shown in figure 6.1. Normal human cells have 46 chromosomes. Two of these are the sex chromosomes and the remaining 44 comprise 22 pairs of somatic chromosomes, one set being inherited from the father and the other from the mother. Cells with this chromosome complement are described as diploid.

It is an almost invariable feature of advanced cancers, particularly solid cancers, that they contain many examples of abnormal karyotypes. Sometimes there is exactly double the normal complement of chromosomes (tetraploid cells) but more commonly the number is somewhere between the diploid and tetraploid number and therefore represents a chromosome imbalance. This condition is called aneuploidy.

In transplanted tumours in experimental animals, the same characteristic phenomenon can be observed. If these tumours are followed through many

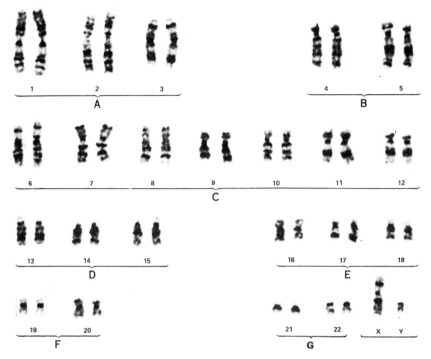

Figure 6.1   Normal human karyotype. (Professor S. Federoff)

generations of transplantation, it is often found that the karyotype changes progressively. Obviously the tumour cells have an instability which is manifested by a propensity for changing their chromosome complement. Whereas in normal cells exactly half of the chromosomes in the dividing cell go to each daughter, in tumour cells the division is often unequal, a condition called non-disjunction. This raises the question whether chromosomal changes are a cause or a result of the cancer process.

From experiments in animals and in isolated cells, it is known that viruses often cause chromosome breaks and that x-rays and some chemicals can also do this. Since all these agents have been implicated as aetiological factors in cancer, it is a plausible hypothesis that damage to the chromosomes or to the mitotic apparatus can initiate cancer and that the cancerous process itself is a consequence of the chromosomal imbalance. However, not all the facts fit with this hypothesis. Many experimental virus-induced tumours show no demonstrable abnormalities of the chromosomes at all in the early stages of transformation and only after the tumours have grown through many passages do the typical progressive karyotypic abnormalities emerge. Similarly, some transformed cells produced by carcinogens do not exhibit chromosome breaks while, on the other hand, chemicals which readily produce chromosome breaks (for example, caffeine) are not known to be carcinogens. Also, though x-rays do cause both chromosome breaks and cancer, there is no clear correlation between the number of chromosome breaks produced and the incidence of cancer.

The study of the cell karyotype is, of course, a rather crude way of looking at genetic changes and the use of more refined methods of analysis may show that genetic damage is more widespread in these instances than would appear to be the case.

In some human cancers, characteristic chromosomal abnormalities appear. In particular, 90 per cent of all cases of chronic granulocytic leukaemia show an abnormality of chromosome 22. This is normally an asymmetric chromosome with one short arm and one long arm. In chronic granulocytic leukaemia (CGL), the long arm is absent, giving rise to what is called the Philadelphia chromosome. However, the Philadelphia chromosome is not present in all mitotic cells in the body in cases of CGL. It occurs only in the haemopoietic system where it can be seen not only in myeloid cells but also in erythroid precursors and megakaryocytes. This chromosomal abnormality occurs so frequently (although not always) in the disease that it is almost certainly meaningful in relation to its causation. In advanced leukaemia, as in other cancers, progressive karyotypic abnormalities eventually emerge but these late changes have no recognisable distinguishing features.

This feature of chronic granulocytic leukaemia appears to be unique and so far nothing corresponding to it has been recognised in any other kind of leukaemia. In some acute leukaemias, gross aberrations of the chromosomes occur. Burkitt's lymphoma, which may be caused by a tumour virus, also shows chromosomal aberrations rather frequently.

HEREDITARY PREDISPOSITION TO CANCER

The chromosomal changes in tumour cells which have been described seem likely to be consequences rather than causes of the disease. However, there is very convincing evidence for a hereditary element in many experimental animal tumours, and it is clear that in some human tumours a hereditary element is involved.

The inheritance of susceptibility to tumours has been quite extensively studied in experimental animals. In the course of cancer research, many strains of mice with a susceptibility to a particular kind of tumour have been identified or bred. The C3H mouse came to prominence as already mentioned because almost all the females develop mammary tumours due to the transmission of the mammary tumour virus from mother to infant in the mother's milk.

Among other mouse strains with inherited tendencies to develop cancer are the BALB/c strain which has a high susceptibility to spontaneous lung tumours, the CBA strain which develops hepatomas and the C58 strain which is prone to develop leukaemia.

Breeding experiments also lead to the conclusion that genetic factors of a general kind may be involved in cancer susceptibility. In two kinds of fish, the platyfish and the swordtail, melanoma tumours are virtually unknown yet in hybrids between them, they occur with a very high frequency. Similarly, in crosses between different strains of mice, tumours are in general rather more frequent in hybrids than in the parents.

These kinds of observations in experimental animals have their parallel in some cancers in man, most of which are rather rare.

Chromosomal abnormalities are a frequent consequence of malignant transformation but from the studies described earlier there is not very strong evidence that they regularly precede cancerous changes. However, there are a number of human diseases which are characterised by chromosomal abnormalities and in which an increased incidence of cancer, particularly leukaemia, is observed.

The most common of these is Down's syndrome or mongolism. This well-known disease is due to the presence of an extra chromosome 21; in these individuals, there are three of these chromosomes instead of the usual pair. Their chromosomal imbalance is sufficient to cause all the stigmata of the disease and one well-known feature of Down's syndrome is an increased incidence of leukaemia. Kleinfelter's disease involves a similar imbalance. In this condition, the individuals have three sex chromosomes (2X and 1Y) instead of two. They also exhibit a higher incidence of leukaemia than normal persons.

Moreover, there is a group of diseases distinguished by a tendency for the chromosomes to be fragmented and which is also associated with a high incidence of cancer. All of these diseases are inherited as genetic recessives and therefore the disease only becomes manifest when the defect is inherited from both parents.

The first of the conditions exhibiting a tendency to spontaneous chromosome breaks is called Fanconi's anaemia. Cells from these patients are exceptionally sensitive to x-rays and to x-ray-induced chromosome breakage. Interestingly enough, fibroblasts from these patients are also particularly susceptible to transformation by the SV40 virus. Patients with Fanconi's anaemia have a quite high probability of dying of leukaemia. Two other rare diseases, Bloom's syndrome and ataxia-telangiectasia, exhibit very similar phenomena. They are both recessive characteristics, show increased chromosomal fragility and pre-dispose to leukaemia. It is suspected that in all these diseases, the underlying lesion is a defect of DNA repair.

In the fourth of these diseases, xeroderma pigmentosum, it has already been remarked that defective repair occurs. The manifestations of this disease are particularly observed in the skin. The sufferers are exceedingly sensitive to sunlight and other forms of irradiation and have a high incidence of skin cancers.

Several other human cancers show an even greater hereditary element in that they are inherited as a dominant characteristic. The best known among these is polyposis coli. The multiple polyps occurring in the colon in this disease have a high likelihood of developing into adenocarcinomas (figure 6.2). These are not the only tumours to which these patients are susceptible for they sometimes have tumours elsewhere, usually of the connective tissues.

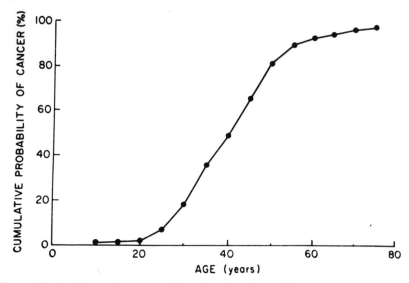

Figure 6.2   Incidence of cancer of the colon in patients with polyposis coli by age. (Fraumeni, J. F. Jr. and Mulvihill, J. J. in *Cancer Epidemiology and Prevention* (Ed. D. Schottenfeld), Thomas, Springfield, Illinois, 1975, p. 405)

The basal cell naevus syndrome is also inherited as a dominant characteristic. This is a complex condition involving skeletal abnormalities, ectopic calcification and epidermal cysts as well as the multiple basal cell carcinomas of the skin which characterise the disease and give it its name.

Some tumours which occur in children have a strong hereditary element. Forty per cent of all retinoblastomas are hereditary. About 40 per cent of Wilm's tumours are also familial and there is a hereditary element in over 20 per cent of neuroblastomas. Other forms of cancer in which hereditary elements are prominent are phaeochromocytomas, neurofibromatosis and the multiple endocrine tumour syndrome, a rather rare condition which is inherited as a dominant characteristic.

All these human cancers in which inheritance is a prominent feature are extremely rare and it should be emphasised that in most of the commoner cancers there is no evidence at all of a genetic element although it is not unlikely that a fraction of all tumours, perhaps a few per cent, may involve an element of hereditary predisposition.

Obvious hereditary disorders like polyposis coli or xeroderma pigmentosum are not the only kinds of diseases which may predispose to cancer.

Table 6.1 Predisposing diseases in human cancer

Tumour	Predisposing disease
Carcinoma of mouth ⎱ Carcinoma of vagina ⎰	Leucoplakia
Carcinoma of oesophagus	Plummer–Vinson syndrome
Carcinoma of stomach	Achlorhydria, pernicious anaemia
Carcinoma of colon	Polyposis coli, ulcerative colitis, Gardner's syndrome
Carcinoma of small bowel	Peutz–Jegher's syndrome, Crohn's disease, coeliac disease
Carcinoma of skin	Fair complexion, xeroderma pigmentosum
Hepatoma	Cirrhosis
Testicular tumours	Cryptorchidism
Leukaemia	Bloom's syndrome, Fanconi's anaemia
Osteosarcoma	Paget's disease
Various	Immunodeficiency disease, idiopathic or acquired

Other chronic conditions like achlorhydria and ulcerative colitis also carry an increased risk although the likelihood that a hereditary element is involved is much less. In some other predisposing conditions, like cirrhosis of the liver, an inherited component is almost certainly absent. Table 6.1 presents a list of diseases which predispose to certain tumours.

7 Immunological and Endocrine Factors

The two best understood immunological mechanisms are those associated with humoral and cellular immunity. Humoral immunity is the production of soluble antibodies against antigens, commonly bacterial toxins. These antibodies appear in the serum as gamma globulins. Our knowledge of cellular immunity has developed as a result of studies of tissue transplantation. Tissues can be transplanted from one part to another of the same individual or between syngeneic individuals, such as identical twins. However, the transplantation of tissue from one individual to a genetically different one almost always results in its rejection. This rejection reaction, the homograft reaction, is a result of cellular immunity and it is mediated through lymphocytes which have become sensitised to the foreign tissue.

Cancers behave like foreign transplants in that, though much weaker antigens, they can set up both humoral and cellular immune reactions. The humoral reactions are of interest because they provide immunological methods for the detection and monitoring of certain kinds of cancer. Cellular immunity to cancers is important because it may be the body's normal reaction to the emergence of abnormal cells. There has recently been much interest in the proposition that malignant transformation occurs quite frequently but that, because of cellular immunity, the cancer cells are normally destroyed in the body – the immunosurveillance theory. It is postulated that cancer only results when cells fail to provoke a sufficiently strong response or, alternatively, the cellular immune response is overcome, resulting in tolerance of the cancer cells.

CANCER ANTIGENS

Antigens are substances, usually proteins, which provoke an immune response. Nearly all proteins are potentially antigenic for adult mammals which have not been previously exposed to them. However, they provoke no response if present at the time when the immune system develops. In mammals this is usually in late foetal life or, in some instances, around or shortly after birth. Why then do cancer cells stimulate an immune response? There seem to be three reasons. Firstly, entirely new antigens are produced in some cases because of the intervention of tumour viruses. Secondly, in some instances, carcinogenic chemicals give rise to modified proteins. Thirdly, embryonic proteins which were no longer being made by the time the immune system was developed are sometimes made again by cancer cells.

Viral antigens are characteristic of the viruses themselves; all tumours associated with a given virus contain the antigens characteristic of the virus. Antigens of this kind are commonly associated with many experimental tumours of animals such as the Rous sarcoma, murine sarcomas, murine leukaemias and cat leukaemia. Their existence in man would provide strongly suggestive evidence for the involvement of viruses in certain tumours but, apart from Burkitt's lymphoma, the evidence for specific antibodies of the types which would characteristically be associated with tumour viruses is not strong.

Tumour-specific antigens associated with chemically-induced tumours behave very differently in that each tumour has its own specific antigen. Even when different tumours are separately induced in the same animal they are immunologically distinct. The immunity is demonstrated by a rejection test. This test is performed by first exposing animals to tumour antigens either by transplantation of a tumour which is subsequently removed surgically or by inoculation with irradiated tumour cells. If the animal has developed an immunity, on re-inoculation with the tumour at a later date, the animal shows a reaction of rejection against it (figure 7.1).

The antigens associated with these phenomena are of great interest in experimental oncology but have proved disappointing in their application to human disease. The third group of antigens, those due to the reappearance of embryonic proteins, are of greater practical importance in relation to the disease in man. The two most important are the carcino-embryonic antigen and α-fetoprotein. Carcino-embryonic antigen is elevated in the blood of patients with carcinoma of the colon. Unfortunately, its value as a diagnostic agent is reduced by the fact that it can also be detected in increased amount in a large number of other conditions. Although unreliable as a diagnostic tool for this reason, it is nevertheless a useful index which can be used for monitoring patients for possible recurrence of the disease.

Alpha-fetoprotein was originally found in association with experimental liver tumours in rodents but the same kind of protein has also been found to be elevated in human hepatomas. Another rather unusual antigen which has been associated with cancer is the 'cancer-basic protein', the nature and role of which is not yet clear.

While soluble antibodies (gamma globulins) are very important in the defence against bacteria and viruses and may prove useful as diagnostic aids or as monitoring indices in cancer, it is not clear whether they play an important part in the body's defence against cancer cells or not. During recent years, most attention has been directed to the cellular immune mechanisms but there is quite good evidence that circulating antibodies may inhibit metastatic spread. For example, in patients with rapidly metastasising melanomas no circulating antibodies against the tumour cells have been found but antibodies of this kind have been demonstrated in patients with non-metastasising melanomas.

The presence of antibodies to cellular antigens can be demonstrated by immunofluorescence. The most direct way to perform this is by chemically coupling a fluorescent substance to immunoglobulin. When fixed cells are treated with this reagent, the location of antigen can be recognised under the fluorescence microscope by the fluorescent antibody which binds to it. Direct coupling of fluorescin to antibody has now largely been replaced by less direct but technically easier methods. By fluorescent antibody techniques, antigens can be located in different components of the cell. Many tumour-associated antigens are situated on the cell surface but some, for example in melanomas, are in the cytoplasm and others, for example the Epstein–Barr nuclear antigen, are located in the cell nucleus.

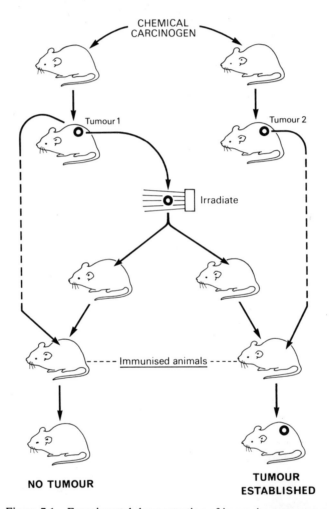

Figure 7.1 Experimental demonstration of immunity to tumours

An entirely different kind of immunity is conferred by interferon. Its mechanism of action is not understood but it provides a general defence against viruses. Production of interferon is stimulated by viral nucleic acids and in its presence viral replication is inhibited.

CELLULAR IMMUNITY

The cells which are concerned with immune responses are all derived from the reticulo-endothelial system. The three kinds of cells which play the most important part in this are lymphocytes, plasma cells and macrophages. It is now recognised that there are at least two different kinds of morphologically indistinguishable lymphocytes, called B cells and T cells. In chickens, B cells are formed in an organ called the Bursa of Fabricius; they roughly correspond to lymphocytes produced in the bone marrow in mammals. Lymphocytes of this kind are mainly involved in the production of antibodies. The T cells are derived from the thymus and are mainly concerned with the process of cellular immunity; when they have been sensitised to certain kinds of cells, they attack and destroy them. In fact, the division between B and T cells is not quite so clear cut as this description would imply and some lymphocytes share characteristics of both B and T cells. The other kind of cell which is involved in the cellular response is the macrophage. It is probably involved in a less highly specific kind of immunity which will be described later.

As discussed above, studies on tumour immunity are based on the observation that inoculation of experimental animals with killed tumour cells endows them with resistance to subsequent inoculation with live cells. The immunity is almost never complete but can be clearly demonstrated by two criteria. The first of these is the number of cells required to produce a tumour. This number varies greatly from one tumour to another. With some of the most virulent experimental tumours in rodents, a single cell or a very few cells will be sufficient to produce a tumour in a susceptible host. With some other transplantable tumours, it is necessary to inoculate with hundreds of thousands or even millions of cells to get a successful take. This observation itself tells us something about the organism's resistance to tumour cells. For each tumour in each experimental system, the inoculum required to produce a tumour is relatively constant but in animals which have been previously inoculated with, for example, irradiated cells, the size of inoculum is greatly increased.

The other criterion is the period between the inoculation and the appearance of the tumour. The factors influencing this are really quite complex but the three main ones are the size of the inoculum, the rate at which the tumour cells grow and the percentage which survive. For a given inoculum, in a standard experimental animal, the latent period is rather constant but in animals which have been inoculated with killed cells, it is greatly extended.

Immunity produced in this way does not appear to be mediated by humoral antibodies but requires intimate contact between lymphocytes and tumour cells (figure 7.2). If the second inoculum of cells is made into a 'privileged' site (a site to which lymphocytes have no access), then the inoculated tumour cells are not susceptible to pre-immunisation of the animal. The brain is an example of such a privileged site as also are artificial perfusion chambers. (These chambers are constructed with membranes which permit

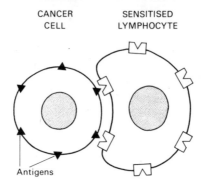

CANCER   SENSITISED
CELL   LYMPHOCYTE

Antigens

Figure 7.2   Diagrammatic representation of recognition of tumour cells by sensitised lymphocytes

free entry of body fluids but exclude cells.) Moreover, this immunity can be abolished by eliminating as far as possible all thymus-derived lymphocytes from the animal. This can be done in several ways, notably by thymectomy of newborn animals or by treating the animals with an antiserum against lymphocytes (antilymphocytic serum: ALS). A strain of mice has also been developed in which the thymus is congenitally absent. These are the so-called 'nude' mice because they lack bodily hair also. All animals which lack thymus-derived lymphocytes are particularly receptive to tumour transplants.

There are, therefore, close parallels between tumour transplantation and normal tissue transplantation. Indeed, the rejection of a foreign tissue by the homograft reaction does involve precisely the same kind of cellular immunity. It has been clearly demonstrated that the rejection and destruction of a foreign tissues and nude mice or immunosuppressed guinea pigs can accept and destroy it. Animals deficient in thymus-derived lymphocytes can tolerate foreign tissues and nude mide or immunosuppressed guinea pigs can accept tissues from entirely different species. There are, however, at least three general differences between transplantation immunity and tumour immunity. The first is that immunity to tumour cells represents an immunity to cells which originated from normal body cells. Secondly, although animals can become resistant to their own tumours, they are, if anything, rather less resistant to transplantation of tumour cells than normal cells from other individuals. Thirdly, the immunity to tumour cells is rather readily overcome when the number of tumour cells exceeds a critical value.

These phenomena have been dissected in some detail by studying them in tissue culture. If cancer cells grown in tissue culture are exposed to lymphocytes from a normal individual, these rarely have a direct effect on the tumour cells. However, if the tumour cells are exposed to sensitised lymphocytes, i.e. lymphocytes from a host immunised against the tumour, then they aggregate round the tumour cells which subsequently die. While sensitised lymphocytes can be particularly easily demonstrated in experimental animals in which tumour immunity has been produced, they can also be demonstrated in certain human tumours. For example, neuroblastoma cells maintained in culture are attacked by lymphocytes from patients with the disease.

It is thought that sensitised lymphocytes recognise antigens on the surface of the tumour cells in much the same way as soluble antibodies recognise the same antigens. However, whereas soluble antibodies are released into the blood, the antibodies in sensitised lymphocytes remain at the cell surface and therefore the lymphocytes must make direct contact with tumour cells in order for the antigens and the antibody (receptor) molecules to interact.

In the neuroblastoma experiments previously mentioned, another phenomenon was discovered. Sensitised lymphocytes from patients in whom the tumour is regressing demonstrate the effect exactly as described above; they attack and kill the tumour cells. But if sensitised lymphocytes are taken from patients in whom the tumour is rapidly progressing, then they exhibit this killing phenomenon only if the patient's own serum is not included in the tissue culture medium. The presence of the patient's serum seems to block the cellular immune response. The serum contains a blocking factor, often referred to as 'blocking antibody'. The term blocking antibody, like many terms used in immunology, is very confusing as its actual nature is not understood. On the one hand, it may be soluble antibody which, by combining with antigens on the surface of cancer cells, blocks them in such a way that the fixed antibodies on the surface of sensitised lymphocytes can no longer attach to them. On the other hand, there is also evidence that they may represent free antigen molecules which block sensitised lymphocytes by attaching to the fixed antibodies on their surfaces. Whatever the mechanism, the important observation is that tumour cells seem to have a mechanism for escaping the host's immunity to the tumour (figure 7.3).

So far the discussion has centred mainly on the role of the thymus-derived lymphocytes in tumour immunity and this is the aspect of tumour immunity which is best understood. However, macrophages are apparently also

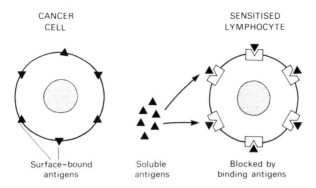

CANCER CELL   SENSITISED LYMPHOCYTE

Surface-bound antigens   Soluble antigens   Blocked by binding antigens

Figure 7.3 Probable mode of action of blocking factors

involved in some kind of cellular immunity. Macrophages express two kinds of activity towards cancer cells. That which is best known is the engulfing and digestion of dead cells. However, macrophages can attack tumour cells in another way, rather like sensitised lymphocytes in that they are directly cytotoxic. There is one apparent difference between the immunity endowed by sensitised lymphocytes and that endowed by activated macrophages in that the lymphocyte immunity is highly specific, that is, it is exhibited only towards tumour cells carrying the specific antigens which have stimulated the immunity. The cytotoxicity exhibited by activated macrophages seems to be much less specific and can even be induced by bacterial toxins.

IMMUNOSUPPRESSION IN EXPERIMENTAL ANIMALS

In view of the demonstrated ability of animals to reject second inocula of tumours, the doctrine of 'immune surveillance' has been proposed. According to this, malignant changes may occur with quite high frequency during the lifetimes of most animals but the emergence of tumours is prevented by the body's immune system. Indeed it has been postulated that this may be the evolutionary reason for the emergence of the mechanism of cellular immunity. This is quite an appealing theory because genetic theory would suggest that at least one cancer cell would arise in every few million cell divisions. Hence, an adult human, which is made of 30 million million cells, might expect to develop cancers several times a year. The fact that this does not happen implies that there is some biological mechanism to prevent it and one suggestion is that cellular immunity provides it. If this were so then it might be expected that, in animals and human beings defective in cellular immunity, tumours would arise more frequently. In fact, as outlined below, this seems to be only partly true.

In experimental animal systems, there is a certain amount of evidence to suggest, as might be expected in view of what has already been said, that cellular immunity plays some part in suppressing tumours. For example, in mice infected with polyoma virus, thymectomy and treatment with antilymphocytic serum gave rise to an increased incidence of tumours. The polyoma virus itself happens to be highly antigenic and cells transformed by polyoma virus produce a very strong tumour specific transplantation antigen (TSTA). Therefore, this may be a rather exceptional case, a conclusion which is perhaps borne out by the fact that similar observations can be made in mice with tumours caused by other viruses, for example, the RNA tumour viruses, whereas the picture is very much less clear cut in relation to tumours caused by chemical carcinogens which give rise to much weaker tumour antigens. There is very little disagreement that treatment of experimental animals with antilymphocytic serum, irradiation or cortisone (all measures which reduce cellular immunity) enhances tumour production by murine sarcoma virus and murine leukaemia virus, whereas there is very little agreement on the conclusions to be reached from similar experiments with tumours induced by chemical carcinogens. There seems to be no increased incidence of methylcholanthrene-induced skin and breast tumours in thymectomised mice and, moreover, in experiments from many laboratories no agreement has been reached about the effect of ALS on the incidence of chemically-induced tumours. Indeed, these experiments have turned up some rather paradoxical results. For instance, ALS-treated germ-free mice do not give rise to any tumours when treated with dimethylnitrosamine while tumours arise in 40 per cent of ALS-treated normal mice when given the same carcinogen.

Generally, similar observations have been made in relation to the natural incidence of tumours in immunosuppressed animals. In strains of mice which carry mammary tumour virus and which have a naturally high incidence of mammary tumours, thymectomy and ALS actually reduce the incidence. Moreover, 'nude' mice show no increased natural incidence of tumours, indeed, they are unusually resistant to certain chemical carcinogens such as methylcholanthrene, dimethylbenzanthracene and benzopyrine.

The general picture which emerges is that extensive immunosuppression in mice does not result in a radically different incidence of tumours (although the spectrum of tumours may vary).

IMMUNOSUPPRESSION IN MAN

There are a number of rather uncommon human conditions in which cellular immunity is either congenitally absent or extensively suppressed and, in patients with these diseases, there is probably a much increased incidence of cancer. However, the findings are by no means conclusive because the reported cases tend to be highly selected and the diagnosis of malignancy, in many cases, is uncertain. The reason for this is that an exceptionally high proportion of the tumours found in humans with immune deficiency are derived from the reticulo-endothelial system itself (i.e. the system concerned with immunity). A particularly high incidence of 'reticulum cell sarcomas' has been reported; although in normal populations this is an extremely rare tumour, it is the commonest tumour among immune-deficient people. On the other hand, it has to be remembered that in this condition there are gross abnormalities of the reticulo-endothelial system. This not only makes histological diagnosis difficult but it also leaves open the question of whether tumours arise in the reticulo-endothelial system in these conditions because the system itself is abnormal or because there is a general absence of immune surveillance.

In most patients receiving organ transplants, particularly kidney transplants, their own immune defences have to be suppressed and in a large series of these patients, there has undoubtedly emerged a much increased incidence of tumours. Again, a very high proportion of these tumours are derived from the reticulo-endothelial system and there is an exceptionally high incidence of reticulum cell sarcomas. On the other hand, certain of the common cancers such as breast cancer are not increased.

Hence, the evidence about the role of cellular immunity in the body's defence against cancer is conflicting. Direct evidence for the occurrence of cellular immunity has been suggested in a large number of human tumours including sarcomas, neuroblastomas, melanomas, carcinomas of the colon and bladder and Burkitt's lymphoma. Cellular immunity may, in fact, play an important part in the elimination of the few cancer cells remaining after the majority have been killed or removed by surgery, radiotherapy or chemotherapy. However, it must be borne in mind that the mechanisms of cellular immunity which have been studied in such detail may not be the only or even the most important defences. If immune surveillance depended solely on the kind of cellular immunity discussed here, then observations of a much higher incidence of all the common tumours in patients in whom it is suppressed would be expected. In this connection, the fact should not be overlooked that cellular immunity of the type discussed is by no means universal. No such system is known in many long-lived marine invertebrates or in plants (including trees which survive for many hundreds of years). Although tumours arise in both of these, they do not occur with a noticeably greater incidence than in mammals. Hence, it seems not unlikely that multicellular organisms have other mechanisms for keeping abnormal growths in check.

HORMONES AND CANCER

We keep returning to the theme that cancer is a breakdown of the social organisation of cells in an organism. Unfortunately, very little is known about the factors which tell cells whether to divide or not and where they should be located. It is assumed that these are chemical messengers of some kind and there is a fair amount of information about one particular group of chemical messengers, the hormones excreted by the endocrine glands. Many, if not all, hormones affect not only the functions of their target tissues but also replication and differentiation of target cells. The most obvious examples are the development of secondary sex characteristics under the influence of the sex hormones. Many target tissues are entirely dependent on the presence of the appropriate hormone and in its absence they may atrophy very extensively. This observation has given rise to the idea that tumours derived from such organs can be profoundly influenced by the appropriate hormones.

This principle was first applied by Beatson in 1895 at a time when nothing at all was known about endocrine glands or hormones. During a prolonged stay in the country, he had noted the use made by farmers of castration and had carefully noted the effects of the secondary sex characteristics. He was particularly intrigued by the relationship which seemed to exist between the ovaries and mammary glands and this led him to perform oophorectomies on women with rapidly growing mammary carcinomas, with noticeable effects on the growth of the cancers. This observation was well ahead of its time but subsequently the general idea has been confirmed by experimental studies in animals and clinical experience in humans. In rats, mammary tumours can be induced by carcinogens. These regularly regress following ablation of either the pituitary gland or the ovaries. However, not all tumours in all species behave in this way. Mammary tumours in mice are quite autonomous and unaffected by removal of pituitary or ovaries. In the human, clinical experience has shown that roughly one third of mammary tumours are hormone responsive; this seems to be correlated with the presence or absence of steroid-receptor proteins in the cells of the tissue.

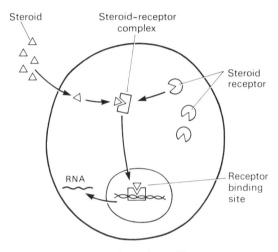

Figure 7.4   Function of steroid receptors

Steroid receptors are proteins which occur in the cytoplasm of target cells but not other cells and have a very high affinity for the steroid molecules. As soon as one of these proteins has bound a steroid molecule, it undergoes a change and almost immediately enters the nucleus and binds to chromosomes. The characteristics of chromosomes are thereby modified in such a way that the spectrum of RNA molecules synthesised in the cell is altered. Most steroid hormones seem to depend on this mechanism but other hormones have other modes of action (figure 7.4).

Since the harmonious functioning of tissues in animals is maintained by hormones, it might not be surprising if serious disturbances of endocrine glands led to cancer and, indeed, in experimental animals this has proved to be the case. The removal of endocrine glands promotes certain tumours. Gonadectomised mice display an exceptional susceptibility to a number of tumours of related organs including oestrogen-secreting adrenal cortical tumours, basophilic pituitary tumours and mammary tumours. The opposite kind of imbalance produced by the sustained administration of hormones can similarly induce tumours and, for example, the prolonged administration of oestrogens in experimental animals gives rise to pituitary tumours which secrete mammotrophic hormone. The prolonged administration of thyrotrophic hormone causes thyroid tumours. Moreover, the blocking of thyroid hormone synthesis by antithyroid substances can also result in thyrotrophic tumours of the pituitary or tumours of the thyroid gland itself.

The effects of hormones in inducing tissue morphogenesis is manifested mainly during embryonic development and very few studies have been undertaken of carcinogenesis at this time. Indeed, it is possible that endocrine malfunctions in early development may have far-reaching effects and one of the most disturbing findings in the human being in recent years has been the observation that daughters of women who received treatment with oestrogens during early pregnancy have an exceptionally high incidence of vaginal carcinomas.

Clinically beneficial effects of endocrine therapy have been reported in many human tumours. Besides cancer of the breast, endocrine therapy has been reported to be of value in cancers of the prostate, thyroid, kidney and endometrium (chapter 15).

8 General Pathology

The preceding chapters have discussed the structure and function of normal cells, some of the abnormalities which distinguish cancer cells and the factors which may be implicated in the disease. It has become evident that cancer is a protean group of disorders with many different manifestations and in the causation of which many different kinds of agents are involved. This chapter discusses the relationships among the different aetiological factors and the common features of cancer which may facilitate the diagnosis of the disease and provide a general basis for its treatment.

PATHOGENESIS

There are three main theories of carcinogenesis:

(1) The viral theory.
(2) The somatic mutation theory.
(3) The epigenetic theories.

The Viral Theory

This is based on experimental work in animals which demonstrates clearly that certain tumour viruses regularly give rise to tumours. In a few instances, such as the Rous virus, cat leukaemia virus and the virus of Marek's disease, direct transmission can readily be demonstrated. Even in these cases, however, the virus does not seem to be the only factor. In experiments in which tissue culture cells are exposed to massive infection with a tumour virus, a relatively small fraction of the cells (a few per cent) undergo the typical transformation and give rise to cells which will subsequently give rise to tumours. The reason for this is not known but it implies that only certain cells, even in a pure population, are susceptible.

Nevertheless, there is a possibility that the virus is a necessary but not sufficient condition for cancer. Some tumour virologists hold this extreme view. How, then, can carcinogenesis by chemicals and x-rays be explained? It is here that the oncogene hypothesis, mentioned in chapter 4, is invoked. In many experimental animals there is indeed evidence that special sequences related to tumour viral sequences are carried in the DNA of all cells and in many experimental situations tumour viruses can be 'rescued' from cells which were not infected by them in the first place. In the human, however, the evidence for involvement of tumour viruses is restricted to Burkitt's lymphoma and warts although there is some suggestion that they may be involved also in certain leukaemias. The present feeling among cancer investigators is that although viruses are necessary for some experimental cancers, they are not necessary for all cancers. Perhaps five per cent of tumours may involve a viral component.

The Somatic Mutation Theory

This theory proposes that all cancers arise as a result of alterations in DNA and there is, indeed, evidence that many may. Now that the facts of molecular genetics are known, it seems certain that some tumours must arise in this way. The problem again is: how many? Currently, it is felt that this is probably rather a high fraction, perhaps as many as ninety per cent. But it is very difficult to reconcile this entirely with the natural history of tumours. Mutations are by definition random events but tumours do not behave in a random and unpredictable way. In fact, the natural history of most tumours is so characteristic that it provides the main basis for diagnosis. Moreover, mutations are rather rare events and one would expect them to give rise to a sudden once and for all change in a cell which would be inherited by its descendants. Tumours, on the contrary, very commonly display a progressive change. The first stage is sometimes a pre-cancerous change which can be recognised before malignancy ensues. Then, as the tumour progresses, the cells often become more bizarre or more primitive. Some very detailed studies have been made of the development of experimental hepatomas in rats, in which the step-by-step loss of specific enzymes has been clearly demonstrated. These observations gave rise to the 'deletion hypothesis' of cancer which proposed that it progresses as a result of the initiation of a chain of events, eventually resulting in the disorganisation of the tissue. It is not easy to reconcile this behaviour with mutation as the sole lesion in cancer.

Epigenetic Theories

These theories are based on the idea that the cancer lesion may not necessarily involve any damage to the genes of the cancer cell but may result from a disruption of the machinery of RNA and protein synthesis which normally determines the differentiated cell. In a way, this is an all-inclusive approach since it could be argued that genetic damage is only one way in which the cell's 'computer' could be disorganised. These theories are formally unsatisfactory because they are not very precise. Therefore it is questionable whether they should be seriously considered at all and we must ask the question: is it possible to demonstrate that cancer cells can revert to complete normality? If they are able to do so, then it can be said that cancer does not necessarily result from an irreversible hereditary change.

The answer is that some tumours can revert to complete normality. Two observations are particularly convincing. The first relates to crown galls, which are tumours in plants. These can be grown in tissue culture and if the cells are treated with the appropriate hormones they can give rise to perfectly normal plants. Plants are a long way from humans and crown galls may have little relevance to human tumours. However, a very similar, though more complicated experiment has been done with mice. It is possible to produce highly malignant teratocarcinomas in mice which are lethal if transplanted to adults. It is also possible in mice to inject a single embryonic cell from one strain into the very early embryo of another strain and to grow these embryos in a foster mother. The mouse which results is a chimera containing cells from both the animal which provided the cell and the animal which provided the embryo. These can be recognised by genetic characterisation. For example, if black and white mice are used the chimera will have black and white stripes. Moreover, by using genetic manipulation, it is possible to ensure that the mouse arising from this operation will be derived only from the single embryonic cell.

Now, when a teratocarcinoma cell instead of a normal embryonic cell is used in this experiment, normal animals result, derived entirely from the tumour cell and having all the genetic characterisations of the animal which gave rise to the tumour.

These experiments convincingly demonstrate that teratocarcinoma cells, if maintained in the appropriate environment, have the capacity to return to complete normality. Interestingly, it is possible that this may occasionally happen with human tumours. Spontaneous regression, though very rare, does occasionally occur. It is generally thought that this is due to immunological rejection but in at least one kind of tumour, neuroblastoma, which regresses with a fair frequency, the suggestion has been made that this recovery is due to normal differentiation of the tumour cells.

It is not easy to reconcile all these observations. Some people argue that cancer is not one disease but includes several kinds of disease. This would provide an easy explanation for the apparently diverse aetiology. However, it is generally felt that all cancers exhibit common features which are related to a common pathogenesis, and this is now thought to be a disturbance of the finely balanced feedback controls which determine cellular differentiation along a specific developmental pathway. The chromosome itself is clearly a particularly vulnerable component of this machinery; hence, it is easy to understand how mutations may play a part. Other vulnerable functions are at present more obscure.

DIAGNOSTIC CHARACTERISTICS OF CANCER CELLS

The definitive diagnosis of most tumours is made by histological study. Tumour histopathology is a very highly specialised art. It requires a detailed knowledge of the normal histology of tissues because cancerous changes, and particularly early cancerous changes, are often recognised only as deviations from normality. Sometimes these are merely subtle changes in tissue architecture such as the disappearance of basal membrane, sometimes they involve recognising anomalies of cells themselves. Indeed, cancer cells do display abnormalities which the skilled eye can sometimes recognise even in isolated cells recovered from effusions.

The most striking features of cancer cells are apparent in the nucleus and, among these, anomalies of mitosis are the most reliable. The occurrence of mitosis in a tissue in which mitosis is rare is suggestive of a malignant change and if the mitotic pattern is grossly abnormal, this can provide very strong evidence. Normal mitosis is bi-polar, that is, the cells contain a single mitotic spindle and the chromosomes divide into two sets, one of which goes to each daughter cell. However, in cancer cells, tri-polar mitoses sometimes occur. The cells have three centrioles and the chromosomes separate into three groups rather than two. Careful study of the chromosomes themselves quite frequently reveals that the karyotype of cancer cells is anomalous. Instead of having the normal diploid complement of chromosomes they may have extra chromosomes or fewer than normal. Within recent years, new techniques have made it possible to recognise a characteristic banded structure in each chromosome. Disturbance of normal banding or evidence that part of a chromosome has been displaced to another chromosome may provide the necessary clue. The above criteria provide very strong evidence of cancerous changes. Some other nuclear changes, which are much less reliable, are fairly commonly associated and may provide useful information for the expert. For example, the nucleus of cancer cells very often exhibits more irregular contours than that of normal cells, the nucleolus is often particularly prominent and the nuclear membrane sometimes appears thicker and more folded.

Often no differences at all can be recognised in the cell cytoplasm but sometimes cancer cells are quite distinctive in that the features of the differentiated cells from which they arose are lost. This loss of special differentiated features is called anaplasia and can be quite extreme so that, for example, cells derived from epithelial cells may have no special features which enable the observer to identify them as being of epithelial origin at all.

Some other grosser features of tumours can also be characteristic. There may be recognisable anomalies of the blood supply and sometimes local haemorrhage although this usually occurs only when a tumour is well developed. Invasion by lymphocytes, macrophages and plasma cells occurs in some cases. However, the most distinctive feature of many malignant cancers is the invasion of adjacent tissues giving rise to the appearance of cancer cells in tissues in which they are never normally found.

More advanced tumours present still more pronounced phenomena. If near a surface, a tumour may break down and become ulcerated. If at all large, it is quite common for the centre to be necrotic because the tumour cells outgrow their blood supply. Stenosis or obstruction may result from the presence of a tumour in a relatively narrow passageway.

PATHOLOGICAL CONSEQUENCES OF TUMOURS

The clinical effects of tumours are caused by their interference with normal function and they can do this in several ways.

Local Disturbance

Many of the symptoms of a tumour arise from the fact that it displaces other tissues; it is a space-occupying lesion. An example of this has been referred to above where the presence of a lump in a narrow tube such as the bronchus or oesophagus may cause obstruction. The main effects of brain tumours are caused by the inability of the skull to accommodate the increased tumour volume with resulting damage to the brain itself.

Metabolic Effects

Some tumours disrupt bodily functions by producing hormones in excessive amounts. For example, the chromaffin tumour (phaeochromocytoma) secretes adrenalin which may cause pronounced symptoms of persistent or paroxysmal hypertension when the tumour is so small that it is extremely difficult to localise it. Similarly, tumours of the Islets of Langerhans may give rise to distressing hyperinsulism although the tumours themselves can only be identified after diligent histological study of the tissue. A more general metabolic change is cachexia, an extreme wasting which occurs in some tumours. At one time, it was thought that this might be due to toxins produced by the cancer but it seems likely that the reasons are more specific. In many cancers anorexia is a prominent symptom and may be the major cause of wasting. In many ulcerating tumours, wasting may be a secondary result of bacterial infection. In a few tumours, the production of ectopic hormones, such as thyrotrophic hormone, may account for loss of weight. It is still not absolutely clear whether cancer may produce some toxins of a specific nature but, on the whole, this is now regarded as unlikely. Indeed, many patients suffering from cancer exhibit no wasting at all.

Metastasis

In many malignant tumours, the fatal effects of the disease are due to a spread of cancer cells. Metastatic spread commonly occurs by five routes – lymphatic, blood-borne, retrograde venous, transcoelomic and invasive. Lymphatic spread is common to most carcinomas. For example, in carcinoma of the breast the tumour cells commonly reach the axillary lymph nodes by way of the lymphatics draining the breast. Blood-borne spread results from local invasion of blood vessels by cells which then become detached and are carried elsewhere. The cells swept along in this way are trapped again when they arrive in a capillary bed, for example, in the lungs, brain or kidneys. Blood-borne cells from the stomach and bowel commonly produce metastasis in the liver, having been carried there by the portal circulation. Retrograde venous spread may be the main explanation for the occurrence of metastasis in the bone marrow. In this instance, the cells are not carried along by the blood stream but actually move back against the general flow, probably because the current in veins without valves can easily be reversed by changes in intra-abdominal or intrathoracic pressure. Transcoelomic spread is a feature of some tumours within the abdominal cavity. Finally, local invasive spread probably represents the fundamental lesion in all metastases.

Part 2

The Clinical Approach to the Patient with Cancer

9 The Approach to the Patient

As with the treatment of any disease the approach to the patient and the attitudes of the doctor or nurse are of crucial importance. This implies that the same high standards of medical care, investigations and treatment are given to the patient with cancer as would be given to other diseases requiring specialist management. It emphasises the fact that the clinical approach to the patient has, as its foundation, the principles of general medicine.

CANCER AS A TREATABLE DISEASE

The first important principle is that the patient with cancer is worth treating, meaning that the cancer patient should be given the same consideration as patients with other illnesses. Certainly treatment is not as simple as it might appear. There are, naturally, situations in which it might be difficult or impossible; it might be associated with severe side effects or, indeed, be unjustified. However, it is important that the clinician does not dismiss all patients with cancer as having untreatable disease.

In this respect it is important to re-emphasise the fact that cancer is not a single disease, but a whole group of diseases. Thus some neoplasms such as squamous carcinomas of the skin are readily treatable with long-term survival figures of over 90 per cent. Others, such as carcinoma of the lung have a much poorer prognosis. It is not possible therefore to lump 'cancers' together. Each must be individually assessed. As will be described later, the outlook for many cancers has changed significantly in the last few years and neoplasms which would previously have been considerably untreatable, are now beginning to yield.

There are many clinicians with a particular interest in the management of the patient with cancer. In this respect the concept of the 'Cancer care team' is important. Just as there are 'Intensive care teams' and 'Coronary care teams' so the patient with cancer should be managed by such an interdisciplinary group. The group would include not only clinicians of varying specialities, but nurses, physiotherapists, medical social workers, pharmacists, basic scientists and many others. Because of the wide range of tumours which may occur, this team approach is essential to bring special expertise to the individual patient. Later in the book the structure of this team is examined in more detail.

The approach to the patient is clearly governed by clinical training and by personal experience of relatives or friends who have had cancer. The fear of cancer is a fear which the professionals also have, and such fears can only be allayed with a knowledge of the progressive advances being made in diagnosis and treatment. The fears of the doctor or nurse, however, may significantly influence the attitude of the patient and his relatives.

COMMUNICATION

In any sphere of medicine, communication is important. In dealing with the patient with cancer, however, this becomes even more crucial. The communication involves not just the patient and the doctor, but associated medical staff, nurses, relatives and ancillary workers.

Communication implies face-to-face contact with the patient; it means getting to know the family and the patient; it means having the time to talk to patients. This is not easy and may involve a great deal of time and effort.

The question always arises as to 'what to tell the patient'. This is an extremely difficult question and might be better put as 'when to tell the patient'. This kind of communication depends a great deal on the patient, the extent of the disease, and on the possibility of effective treatment. The decision to tell a patient requires fine judgement and clearly depends on the skill of the individual doctor and on his assessment of the patient. It has been said that patients should never be told that they have cancer. This view, however, is changing and more and more patients are now aware of the diagnosis. This has not overtly increased the problems associated with managing patients with cancer and indeed it has often made things easier. There is no doubt, however, that the time must be right for such discussions and that the patient must be given a great deal of support following the interview. It is the experience of many groups that when the patients know the diagnosis and understand the reasons for treatment, and the signs and symptoms which they may have, then the management of such patients is facilitated.

The 'conspiracy of silence' which often surrounds the patient with cancer makes communication within the family group difficult and may set up a barrier between the patient and the doctor. Communication with the patient about the type of treatment to be given will also be necessary. The purpose of the operation and its side effects; the problems with drug therapy and the length of the period of treatment; the length of treatment course with radiotherapy. All these questions should be anticipated and answered.

Effective communication between medical specialists and between the hospital and general practitioner services is essential. The same 'story' must be told on each occasion or the patient may rapidly lose confidence in his medical attendants. The nursing staff must also be brought into the communication circle. Their contact and rapport with the patient is an essential part of the overall care of the patient. Other ancillary staff such as social workers and health visitors must also be made fully aware of the patient's knowledge and reaction to the diagnosis.

The relatives must not be forgotten. Not only should they in most instances be informed of the diagnosis and prognosis, but also of the type of treatment to be given and its side effects. At the time of bereavement the relatives must always be remembered. It is often helpful to discuss the treatment plan with the patient and relatives together. Thus each partner becomes more fully aware of the prognosis and no 'secrets' exist between them. This procedure often brings out into the open the specific problems faced by the patient and his relatives.

THE DIAGNOSIS

As with any medical problem it is essential that the diagnosis is established. The definitive evidence required is the histological or cytological confirmation of the clinical findings. This may inevitably mean a bronchoscopy in the elderly or a difficult biopsy. However, modern management of the patient with cancer depends on an accurate diagnosis and competent histology. In difficult cases a discussion of the diagnosis with the pathologist and a review of all pathological material will usually overcome any problems.

Should a patient ever be treated for cancer without a histological diagnosis? In some cases of course it will be difficult to obtain a biopsy either because of technical problems in obtaining material or because the patient is too ill. In these cases the clinical findings must be accepted. However, it should be remembered that once the diagnosis of cancer is made and treatment commenced, the patient is then branded henceforth with the 'cancer stigma'. It should be pointed out that a gastric tumour might be a lymphoma, that every chest shadow is not lung cancer, and that the clinical presentation of chronic pancreatitis may be very similar to that of pancreatic cancer.

It is also important that the same criteria are accepted in the diagnosis of secondary spread. It is a simple matter to assume that the patient with cancer, presenting with new symptoms or signs has developed metastatic disease. However, this attitude of 'guilty till proven innocent' may lead to mistaken diagnoses. It should always be remembered that *'sinister symptoms are sometimes simple'*; that patients with cancer may get headaches, constipation or influenza, and that this may not indicate cerebral secondaries, bowel obstruction or chest metastases. It is essential that application of the principles of diagnosis which would be used in any other medical problem be applied to the cancer patient. It is so easy to assume metastatic disease and to forget that every symptom may not be sinister.

Thus, emphasis is placed on the accuracy of the initial diagnosis as it is on this basis that subsequent treatment decisions will be made. At the present time there is no simple or rapid technique for diagnosing cancer. Clearly it would be of great benefit if a blood test were available for diagnosis. Naturally, many tests have been suggested. They include the measurement of specific and non-specific proteins; DNA binding protein in serum; polyamines in urine; the measurement of serum enzymes including lactic dehydrogenases, glycoprotein transferases; immunological tests of lymphocytes and macrophages, including macrophage electrophoretic migration tests (MEM), and the structuredness of the cytoplasmic matrix (SCM) test. Several fetoproteins including carcino-embryonic antigen (CEA) and α-fetoproteins have also been used for the diagnosis of specific cancers. Although many of these tests are promising, none as yet can be confidently used in the clinical situation for the purposes of diagnosis.

The diagnosis, therefore, must be based on the traditional methods of history taking, physical examination and biopsy or cytology. Investigations including radiology, isotope scanning techniques and ultrasonography will be necessary in the majority of cases.

PREPARATION FOR TREATMENT

Having established the diagnosis several questions must be asked before starting treatment. These include:

(1) Is the cancer localised or has it spread?
(2) What are the patient's main symptoms?
(3) How has treatment to be assessed?

TUMOUR SPREAD – STAGING

The question of staging is an important one in the modern management of the cancer patient. Staging is an attempt to establish, as far as it is possible, whether or not the tumour is localised or has spread. The clinical basis for staging is the principle that localised tumours require local forms of treatment, but when the disease has spread then systemic forms of treatment are necessary. Staging depends on the particular type of tumour and the ease with which it can be detected. With some forms of neoplasm it is impossible to be confident that the tumour is localised, in others this is not the case. The type of tumour also dictates the natural history of the disease and its mode of spread. Squamous carcinomas of the head and neck, and carcinomas of the bladder tend to infiltrate locally and distant spread occurs late. Others such as carcinoma of the lung or breast spread widely.

Two examples may be given to illustrate the value of staging. Hodgkin's disease is a tumour which is particularly responsive both to radiotherapy and chemotherapy. In the typical case presenting with a lump in the neck the prevention of recurrence in that area can be achieved in the majority of patients by regional radiotherapy. It is imperative, however, to be sure that the tumour is localised in the neck. To answer the question properly it is necessary to consider a logical routine of investigations which may include most of the following: a chest x-ray, bone marrow aspiration, lymphangiogram, liver and spleen scan, and possibly a laparotomy with liver biopsy and splenectomy. Such a thorough staging procedure should establish whether the patient has localised disease or disseminated disease which may then be treated accordingly. The value of such a procedure, costly and hazardous as it is, must be justified. In Hodgkin's disease it can be justified by the fact that such a procedure alters the patients clinical staging in over 25 per cent of cases. It has, in addition, allowed a much greater insight into the spread of the disease and in its natural history.

Breast cancer is another type of neoplasm in which staging procedures have altered the treatment policy. Thus the patient who presents with a malignant lump in the breast, may or may not have palpable axillary lymph nodes. Whether they are palpable or not, it is likely that the clinician will be wrong 50 per cent of the time as to node involvement with tumour. In a similar way a skeletal survey will detect only a few patients with bony metastases at the time of diagnosis. Using isotope scanning techniques up to 20 per cent of patients with apparently localised breast cancer will have bone involvement. And, as the sophistication of the investigative techniques increases, then the number of patients with 'early' breast cancer who have distant spread will increase. These facts about breast cancer staging indicate firstly, that clinical techniques alone are not sufficient for adequate assessment, and, secondly, how adequate staging can change the method of treatment, a localised tumour being treated by surgery alone while systematised disease is treated with systemic therapy in addition to removal of the primary tumour.

From these two examples two general questions may be asked.

(1) Why is staging not carried out in all types of neoplasm?

(2) If staging procedures show that many patients have occult disease, why not treat *all* patients with systemic forms of therapy?

The answer to the first question depends on a knowledge of the natural history of the disease, how it spreads and how early the tumour can be detected. If invasive techniques are required then clinicians are often unwilling to submit a patient with apparently localised disease to hazardous investigations. In other instances it is realised that control of the primary tumour will not be possible and that attempts to identify spread of the disease would not alter treatment. In spite of these comments it would seem reasonable that, where possible, investigations should be carried out to determine the full extent of the disease.

To answer the second question is far more difficult. It depends on two factors: the availability of effective systemic therapy against the particular tumour and the acceptability of this treatment in terms of side effects to the patient who may be feeling extremely well. Recently chemotherapeutic regimes have become available for the treatment of several tumour types. These drugs have been shown to be active in patients with advanced disease, and have then been used on patients who have only minimal amounts of tumour. However, in some tumour types the evidence is not yet available which would make the use of drugs in early disease, or in all patients, a feasible proposition. The problem, of course, is side effects and this will be discussed at length later. However, it is not too early to note that the rational use of chemotherapy in selective situations has altered the outlook for several tumour types, and it is to be hoped that the number of patients who will benefit from this will increase.

SYMPTOMATOLOGY

There is little point in making a diagnosis of cancer and, by sophisticated techniques, establishing the spread of the disease without actually listening to the patient and identifying his complaints. These may vary from pain to dyspnoea, cough, dysuria, insomnia or anorexia. The patient will expect that these symptoms will be relieved by treatment. If effective anti-tumour treatment can be given, and the symptoms are related to the cancer, then these should be relieved. However, this may not always be the case either because therapy is ineffective or because the treatment may take time to alleviate the symptom. In either event it is important that specific symptoms, especially pain, are relieved as soon as possible. To have a good sleep at night and a pain-free day will make the patient feel better and much more able to cope with treatment problems. Many symptoms, notably the troublesome weakness and anorexia often complained of by patients, are difficult to control. In this situation the support and comfort offered by the cancer care team may be invaluable. Once again it is emphasised that every symptom which the patient has may not be sinister and that other causes for any symptoms should be excluded.

SUPPORTIVE THERAPY PRIOR TO TREATMENT

In the initial investigation of the patient it may become apparent that prior to commencing treatment of the tumour, other forms of therapy may be required. These may include blood transfusion to correct anaemia, the use of vitamin supplements and/or parenteral nutrition prior to extensive surgery, or the control of infection. Thus the patient with oesophageal cancer may require blood transfusions and, if dysphagia has been a problem, parenteral nutrition given prior to operation will improve healing of the anastomoses and the wound. In other situations, notably the leukaemias, it is important that infection, however trivial, is recognised and controlled prior to the institution of therapy.

THE EVALUATION AND ASSESSMENT OF TREATMENT

It is an important principle of cancer care that whatever treatment is used the results of that treatment be assessed. This does not imply that all patients with cancer should be involved in controlled clinical trials but it does mean that prior to treatment sufficient information on the extent of the disease spread should be available, in order that the therapy used can be evaluated. Thus obvious disease can be recorded and the effect of treatment monitored. This would allow the therapy to be altered at the earliest possible time when tumour recurred or progressed. In addition to standard radiological, biochemical and haematological measurements, the measurement of biological markers released by tumours should be considered.

Biological markers are substances present within, or released by, neoplasms which can be sequentially measured in blood or urine and allow monitoring of cancer growth (see table 2.2). The measurement of such substances and their change with treatment often gives a very good idea as to the effectiveness of therapy. Choriocarcinoma is a rare tumour which occurs following pregnancy. It releases into the urine, human chorionic gonadotrophin which can be readily measured, and the level of this hormone is related to the tumour mass. Progress can be readily monitored by sequential urinary analysis.

Another group of substances are the oncofetal proteins such as carcino-embryonic antigen (CEA) and α-fetoprotein. Initially the measurement of these compounds was thought to be useful in the early detection of cancer, particularly of the gastrointestinal tract. However, this has proved not to be as worthwhile as originally thought. These compounds, however, are of considerable value in the follow up of patients with various types of cancer. It is essential that a pre-treatment level is obtained, as not all patients may have elevated levels present in serum at the time of diagnosis.

For the patient with advanced disease it is just as important to measure the extent of the disease as it is in patients with early tumours. The size of each lesion should be accurately recorded and measured serially. Only in this way can objective evidence of response to therapy be obtained. If a patient is going to respond to treatment, e.g. with radiotherapy, chemotherapy, or hormone therapy, then it is likely that this will be apparent within two months. The corollary to this is that if the patient has *not* responded in this time it is essential to review therapy. Three situations can be visualised and a decision regarding management made on the basis of the type of response.

(1) Progression of disease, clearly evident by the general condition of the patient or enlargement of the tumour. In this case treatment should be changed or, if the patient's general condition warrants it, stopped altogether.

(2) Regression of tumour, measured objectively. In this circumstance treatment should be continued and reviewed again in a further 2–3 months.

(3) Stable disease, no evidence of progression or regression. In this situation, provided the treatment is not having severe side effects it should be continued but reviewed in 2–3 months. If an alternative treatment is available it should be considered at this point.

The importance of accurate assessment of the status of the tumour cannot be overstressed. It prevents needless treatment where it is ineffective, and allows early institution of other forms of therapy which might be beneficial.

During the follow up of patients careful records should be kept and documentation of changes in treatment or disease status accurately noted. Discharge summaries from hospital, death certificates and other official documents require special care in completion. The data obtained from such documents is used to compute incidence rates and mortality statistics and these are essential tools for the epidemiologist.

REHABILITATION AND TERMINAL CARE

Rehabilitation is a word not often associated with cancer, yet it plays an important part in the management of many types of tumour. It encompasses not only physical, but also psychological and social rehabilitation. Physical rehabilitation includes the encouragement and expertise necessary to maintain or regain organ function following treatment. The amputation of a limb is a good example of how with the proper equipment and care, the patient may walk again and return to a normal life. Speech therapy following partial or complete removal of the tongue or larynx is another example. Paraplegic patients with a potentially recoverable lesion require intensive care to prevent contractures, skin problems and muscle wasting during the period of immobility.

Psychological rehabilitation can be more difficult. Following mastectomy, the patient may have great difficulty in adjusting to a normal life style and may find relationships with her husband very difficult. Careful pre-operative preparation is required, followed by post-operative support and help. Speech difficulties or unsightly scars may also pose problems which, if handled appropriately, can gradually be overcome.

Likewise, social problems can be difficult to solve. The return of the housewife to look after the family after a serious illness or the return of the breadwinner to his employment are often fraught with difficulties. If anticipated and raised with the patient then the problem can often be sorted out before trouble starts.

Terminal care is a part, not only of cancer care, but of the general medical care of any patient. Yet as a subject it is often identified with cancer. The approach of the clinician to the terminal patient will be detailed later, but at this stage it is important to state that terminal care is an active process requiring as much time and careful thought as any other part of management. It is inadequate to relegate the patient to the end of the ward or forget about him just because the time for active anti-tumour treatment is over. That is the time when active symptomatic treatment should begin.

10 Diseases Associated with Cancer

Because cancer can occur in any organ of the body, it is not surprising that the presentation of cancer can be both predictable and unpredictable. In a similar way the patient with cancer may be subject to a wide variety of disease states which have become associated with neoplasms. Such associated problems may be related to the effects of the tumour, either primary or secondary, or to the effects of treatment of the cancer. This chapter, therefore, is concerned with host–tumour relationships, and discusses the effects of the tumour on the patient, and the response of that patient to his disease. Psychological aspects of cancer, pain and immunological aspects of neoplasia are considered elsewhere and are an integral part of this relationship.

BIOCHEMICAL EFFECTS OF NEOPLASIA

One of the most striking features of advanced malignant disease is cachexia. This is a symptom complex associated with tiredness, anorexia, weakness and loss of weight. At a biochemical level various abnormalities have been defined though none can be considered characteristic. There is loss of body fat and protein, the basal metabolic rate may be increased, and there is often an associated peripheral oedema of complex aetiology. Cachexia is a troublesome problem, the weakness and anorexia having a profoundly disturbing effect on the individual. Treatment is unsatisfactory. Corticosteroids and anabolic steroids have been used. The role of elemental nutrition and parenteral feeding remain to be elucidated.

A further broad group of biochemical problems relates to the secretion by the tumour of ectopic hormones (table 2.5). These hormones are synthesised by the neoplasm and have the same systemic effects as naturally occurring products. Thus ACTH secretion produces a cushingoid facies, osteoporosis, hypokalaemia etc. The secretion of antidiuretic hormone (ADH) by cancers causes water retention with a dilutional hyponatremia and associated neurological problems. There is increasing recognition of the release of such products by tumours and the list of proven ectopic hormone secretion now includes MSH, TSH, insulin, glucagon, gastrin, parathormone. Treatment is directed at eliminating the neoplasm since, if this is successful, the symptoms and signs of ectopic secretion are usually abolished. Where this is not possible supportive care is necessary to relieve symptoms. Thus with the ADH secreting tumours, water restriction or hypertonic saline may be required.

There are many other biochemical problems related to tumours. Repeated vomiting or intestinal obstruction may result in severe electrolyte imbalance. Diarrhoea, especially if associated with breakdown of colonic mucosa or a villous papilloma may cause severe hypokalaemia. Involvement of liver or kidney inevitably results in biochemical abnormalities. Rapid tumour breakdown, or cell kill, may result in hyperuricaemia. This may also be related to treatment. More recently the trace metals zinc and copper have been recognised as having important biochemical functions in cancer patients.

One of the most common biochemical problems is hypercalcaemia. This is most often the result of active bone destruction by the tumour and may be related to prostaglandin activity. It may also be related to immobilisation or, more rarely, to ectopic secretion of parathyroid hormone. The symptoms of hypercalcaemia are related to the effects of calcium on the kidneys, brain and gut. It causes polyuria and polydypsia because of its action on the kidneys. Intestinal effects of high serum calcium include anorexia, nausea and vomiting. The effect on the central nervous system is to induce changes in mood and in consciousness level progressing to coma. Treatment is by fluid replacement, usually with saline, and the addition of phosphates, corticosteroids or calcitonin. Several chemotherapeutic agents have been reported to reduce the serum calcium. These include mithramycin and Actinomycin D. The most effective method, however, is to deal specifically with the tumour.

DERMATOLOGICAL EFFECTS OF CANCER

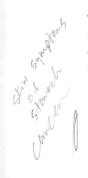

The skin is often said to reflect the internal environment of the body. It does so in many other forms of illness, including gastrointestinal and rheumatic diseases. Cutaneous manifestations of cancer are perhaps more common than is usually recognised, though individually they may be rare. In some cases the presentation of the patient with a skin disorder may alert the physician to look further for internal malignancy.

For example dermatomyositis, and acquired icthyosis occur in lung, breast, and gastrointestinal neoplasms, and lymphomas. Disorders of pigmentation include acanthosis nigricans and addisionian pigmentation. Perioral pigmentation occurs in the Peutz–Jegher's syndrome. A variety of erythematous conditions occur: telangectasia, thrombophlebitis, erythroderma. The endocrine associated tumours produce skin manifestations, such as hypertrichosis, cushingoid facies, gynaecomastia and acne. Pruritus and herpes zoster are two additional skin manifestations of cancer.

MUSCULOSKELETAL EFFECTS OF CANCER

Dermatomyositis and hypercalcaemia have already been mentioned. The muscle weakness in cachexia should not be confused with the more specific myopathies which occur. These include myositis, which is characterised by an inflammatory reaction in muscle, clinically presenting as weakness of proximal muscles. Muscle necrosis occurs and is accompanied by elevated lactic dehydrogenase and creatinine kinase levels in serum. The myasthenic syndrome (Eaton–Lambert syndrome) is a symptom complex very like true myasthenia, but differs pharmacologically and electromyographically. The proximal muscles are affected and have a poor response to neostigmine. Guanidine has been used for treatment.

The skeletal effects of cancer are related predominantly to bone destruction, though osteoporosis can occur. Bone destruction by cancer can manifest itself radiologically as lytic areas or as areas of increased density, osteosclerotic metastases. These areas may be detected by the use of skeletal scintiscans before radiological changes are noted. Clinically the metastases are often associated with pain, and fractures through fragile bone may occur. Mechanisms of bone destruction are being investigated at present and there is some evidence that prostaglandins are involved. Because of the pharmacological interaction between prostaglandins and aspirin, bone pain may often be relieved by the use of salicylates. Radiotherapy to the area is often very effective in relieving pain. For stabilisation, pinning of the fracture may be required. When bone lesions are multiple, systemic therapy is necessary.

NEUROLOGICAL EFFECTS OF CANCER

As with the other effects described neurological problems may arise without direct invasion of the nervous system by the tumour. Carcinomatous neuropathy is a term which includes a chronic distal polyneuropathy and a carcinomatous sensory neuropathy. In contrast, the myelopathy associated with cancer is relatively rare. Subacute cerebellar degeneration presents clinically with ataxia, instability of gait and dysarthria, without evidence of tumour involvement in the posterior fossa. Several forms of encephalopathy have been associated with cancer. Most of these are very rare. Progressive multifocal leukoencephalopathy, though rare, is of some interest as it may be related to virus infection.

HAEMATOLOGICAL EFFECTS OF CANCER

Haematological complications of cancer are relatively common, and occur not only in relation to tumour growth but as a result of treatment.

Anaemia

Anaemia may occur for many reasons, some of which are listed below.

(1) Marrow infiltration by tumour. This may occur without bone destruction. The marrow elements are gradually replaced by malignant cells and the peripheral blood film may show evidence of immature cells (leukoerythroblastic anaemia).

(2) Marrow fibrosis. This may be haematologically very similar to marrow invasion. Bone marrow examination is essential to confirm the diagnosis.

(3) Blood loss. This occurs in a wide variety of neoplasms.

(4) Effects of treatment. Chemotherapy and radiotherapy both have a direct effect on bone marrow. Surgical removal of parts of the gastrointestinal tracts, e.g. stomach, terminal ileum, may result in megaloblastic anaemias.

(5) Malabsorption. This occurs in some patients with cancer and affects not only iron absorption but vitamin B12 and folate.

(6) Non-specific factors. A moderate anaemia, the anaemia of 'chronic inflammation', may occur in patients with cancer and for whom the above factors can be excluded. Many hypotheses have been proposed to account for these facts though none, as yet, fully explain the mechanism.

(7) Haemolytic anaemias. In various neoplastic diseases, haemolysis may occur, related to an immune phenomenon. The Coomb's test is frequently positive in such patients. In others cold agglutinins may be present. Microangiopathic anaemia, characterised by red cell distortion and fragmentation, has been described in patients with widespread cancer.

(8) Pure red-cell aplasia is rare and may be associated with a thymoma.

Platelets

For similar reasons platelet levels in peripheral blood may be reduced considerably. The low platelet count is particularly life threatening because of the danger of bleeding. Not only is platelet production decreased because of marrow involvement or anti-cancer therapy, but platelets are destroyed during intravascular coagulation, and other haematological complications. In some instances, notably in myeloproliferative disorders associated with malignancy, platelet counts may rise considerably. This thrombocytosis is associated with increased risk of thrombosis.

White Cell Function

The total leucocyte count may vary greatly in the cancer patient, in addition to that observed in the haematological malignancies. Leucocytosis may occur in infection, and leucopenia may be due to marrow involvement, or the effects of therapy. The problem is that host defences are reduced when the white cell count is low, and there is an increased risk of infection. When the lymphocyte count is reduced the immune response may be depressed.

Disseminated Intravascular Coagulation

This may occur in conditions other than cancer. It is characterised by the activation of the plasma coagulation system. There is deposition of platelet clots within the microcirculation which results in a rapid consumption of coagulation factors such as fibrinogen, and at the same time the platelet count falls, accelerating the process. Clinically the most important feature is haemorrhage, which may occur throughout the body. The control of the problem is difficult but supportive haematological care, the control of sepsis, and the use of heparin may all be required. Other coagulation problems occur in patients with cancer. These include superficial thrombophlebitis and deep venous thrombosis. Prior to operative treatment the cancer patient should always be considered for prophylactic anticoagulation or other methods for the prevention of deep venous thrombosis.

HAEMATOLOGICAL SUPPORT FOR CANCER PATIENTS

From the above comments it will be clear that the need for blood components is often necessary during the management of cancer. Many of the chronic problems can be anticipated and corrected as appropriate. For example, following operations on the gastrointestinal tract, or where malabsorption is evident, haematological problems may be prevented. In a similar way, when radiotherapy and chemotherapy are used, haematological complications can often be predicted and corrected. Blood components, red cells, platelets and leucocytes may be required together or individually. Whenever they are required a clear indication must be present, and an understanding of their usefulness is essential.

Red Cell Transfusions

This may be necessary because of blood loss or because of the use of chemotherapy or radiotherapy inhibiting red cell replacement. Whole blood, or packed cells are usually given. Blood should be screened for the presence of hepatitis-associated antigen. Occasionally, where the possibility of leucocyte transfusions or bone marrow transplantation is being considered, washed red cells, free of HLA antigens should be used.

Platelet Transfusions

Platelet transfusions may be required to control severe bleeding related to a low platelet count. This may be secondary to antineoplastic therapy, or related to disseminated coagulation. Platelets are removed from freshly donated blood and are usually given in the form of concentrates. As platelet viability decreases rapidly with storage it is essential that they are given as soon as possible after collection. The average adult will require four units of platelets to increase the platelet count, post transfusion, by 20 000/mm³. In the presence of infection or other complicating factors this figure may not be reached. Where transfusion reactions occur HLA-type platelets may be required. There is no doubt that the introduction of platelet transfusions has decreased the mortality rate in the acute leukaemias by the reduction in the incidence of fatal haemorrhage. It has been recommended that when the platelet count is less than 20 000, even in the absence of bleeding, platelet transfusions should be given prophylactically.

White Cell Transfusions

While the introduction of platelet transfusions has reduced the mortality from haemorrhage, the use of leucocyte transfusion is under study for the treatment of infection associated with leucopenia. The collection of leucocytes may be from patients with chronic myeloid leukaemia, or from normal donors using the cell separator. This machine is able to separate white cells from the red cell component of the blood. These cells may then be stored and retransfused into the leukaemic patients during episodes of leucopenia. HLA matched leucocytes may also be given to patients with severe depression of the peripheral white count.

Bone Marrow Transplantation

This form of haematological support may be necessary in relation to treatment problems such as an acquired aplastic anaemia. It may also be used in a planned manner in the treatment of some forms of cancer. In this case the bone marrow and the tumour are deliberately destroyed using a combination of cytotoxic drugs and radiotherapy. When this has occurred the patient is transplanted with normal, usually HLA matched bone marrow. This procedure is currently at the developmental stage.

INFECTION AND THE CANCER PATIENT

Cancer patients seem particularly prone to develop infections. Indeed 36 per cent of all cancer deaths are related to infective complications. Many factors, such as those listed below, are responsible for this increased risk of infection.

(1) Presence of metastatic disease, e.g. in lung or urinary tract, predispose to local infection.

(2) Presence of neutropenia, either because of marrow invasion or because of chemotherapy or radiotherapy.

(3) Depression of the immune response. This occurs in advanced cancer and is related to a defect in cellular immunity. In those haematological neoplasms which have abnormalities of the immunoglobulins, infection may also occur.

Although the majority of infections are localised in origin, there is a higher than normal proportion of unusual infections. These include not only bacterial but fungal and viral diseases. The clinician must be constantly on his guard against the development of rare infections. In the severely ill or leucopenic patient on immunosuppressive drugs, these may not present with the classical features of infection. Fever may be absent, there may be no leucocytosis and an absence of localising signs and symptoms. They·may often only be diagnosed by the increased awareness and alertness of the clinician. Confirmation of the causal organism is essential, and all attempts should be made to culture the organism and define its sensitivity to antibiotics. Blood cultures, cultures of sputum, urine, faeces and CSF may all be essential. In the case of chemotherapy which is intended to make the patient leukopenic for a prolonged period (e.g. in the acute leukaemias) then regular culturing of urine, sputum, faeces, and the taking of nasal, aural, throat, axillary and inguinal swabs is essential to monitor changes which occur in the bacterial flora.

When severe infections do occur in leukopenic patients they require aggressive therapy with the appropriate antibacterial agents, supplemented as required by leucocyte transfusions. The organisms involved may be gram negative rods, and a broad spectrum of antibiotic activity should be used in the first instance. As these patients may also have low platelet counts, intramuscular injections should be avoided to prevent haematomas. In the patient who has non-specific signs and symptoms, or may be generally unwell, the presence of tuberculosis should be considered.

Fungal infections are becoming increasingly recognised in the patient with advanced cancer or in whom chemotherapy has been used. Candidiasis is the most common and may be disseminated. Aspergillosis, cryptococcosis and nocardiasis all occur and require aggressive treatment. Protozoal infections with pneumocystis carinii or toxoplasmosis must also be considered. Viral infections are more difficult to treat, but an attempt should be made to make the correct diagnosis.

In the neutropenic patient who becomes febrile it is essential that treatment is started as soon as possible with a range of drugs which will cover all eventualities. Such an aggressive approach has resulted in a diminution of mortality. In the patient who is neutropenic but does not have an infection, therapy may be considered. The patient is given antibiotics to sterilise the gut, placed on sterile food, and nursed in a sterile environment, either a room or a laminar flow hood. Such regimes reduce the infection problem but can usually only be instituted in specialised units.

11 The Management of Cancer

In the past few years there have been considerable changes in methods of treating cancer. These changes have not simply been due to improvements in techniques or the availability of new drugs. The changes have also been related to the way in which the different forms of treatment have been used. For example, the active and aggressive treatment of small amounts of residual tumour, and the concept of combined modality therapy in which the patient may receive several forms of treatment given in a planned manner.

MEASUREMENT OF RESPONSE TO TREATMENT

In the assessment of any form of treatment it is essential that there is some objective method of measuring response. In the cancer patient, objective responses are usually measured by an estimation of the size of the primary lesion or of a metastatic deposit. Following treatment the tumour may respond in several ways.

(1) Complete response. This indicates complete disappearance of all measurable tumour.

(2) Partial response. In this case the tumour mass decreases by at least 50 per cent when measured objectively.

(3) Stable response. No change in the size of the lesion.

(4) Progression. Increase of at least 25 per cent in the size of the tumour.

It should be realised that in many cases it may be extremely difficult to measure such a response. The vague epigastric mass of a neoplasm of the stomach cannot readily be quantified, nor can barium meal examinations. However, the fact that it may be difficult to perform is no excuse for not attempting an objective assessment of therapy. In subsequent sections the 'response rates' include both partial and complete responses.

It is necessary to distinguish between objective responses and symptomatic responses. The relief of pain or the increase in well-being of the patient may be achieved without any clear effect on the tumour being noted. These effects are extremely important to the patient but they may be due to many factors, other than specific anti-tumour therapy. Symptomatic responses should be reported separately. When treatment has been instituted it is necessary to assess its effectiveness at regular intervals. In the case of chemotherapy or radiotherapy the review would be made at 2–3 months after initiation of therapy. At this time the response – complete, partial, stable or progression – would be assessed and a management decision taken as to whether therapy should or should not be continued. Review sessions form an important part of the management of the cancer patient.

Prognostic Factors

When any particular tumour is considered, prognostic factors can often be identified. Such factors can be shown either to alter survival rates or to modify the response to treatment. The menopausal status in patients with breast cancer is an example of an important prognostic factor. The type of histological appearance in lung cancer, oat cell, anaplastic, adenocarcinoma, or squamous cancer, significantly affects the survival rate and response to therapy. The age of the patient, extent of disease, previous treatments, and disease-free interval may all be important. These prognostic factors should be considered when clinical trials are being designed to assess the effect of treatment. Stratification into groups which have similar prognostic factors is essential if the trial is to have any meaning.

Clinical trials remain amongst the most powerful methods for improving the treatment of the patient with cancer. The construction of these trials is therefore crucial and, in addition to establishing carefully stratified groups according to prognostic factors, attention should be given to the method of assessing response. It is particularly important that a limited number of questions are asked in the clinical trial, and that the trial has sufficient patients to answer these questions.

One factor which is correlated with the outcome of treatment is the performance status of the patient. This status gives a numerical value to the overall clinical picture of the patient. Several methods have been used. The Karnovsky Index gives the patient a percentage score: 100 per cent meaning that the patient is very well, 0 per cent meaning death, and intermediate scores indicating a range of patient activity. The Eastern Co-operative Oncology Group have devised the following simple scoring system.

0 – Patient very well, no symptoms.

1 – Patient well, symptoms present, less than normal activity, but not interfering with work and not sufficient for the patient to be in bed.

3 – Patient in bed, but able to get up to toilet. In bed less than 50 per cent of the time.

4 – Patient has severe symptoms, in bed more than half the time.

Such a scoring system, while not adding to a general clinical impression, does allow the patient to be followed at intervals, and statements made as to improvement in performance, and hence the quality of life of the cancer patient.

THE PRINCIPLES OF MANAGEMENT OF THE PATIENT WITH CANCER

It is now possible to summarise the principles which have been outlined in this section of the book. It is essential that the patient should be treated as a whole and that all his needs, physical, psychological, social and spiritual be adequately examined and fulfilled as required. It is considered important that the patient is cared for by a team of motivated clinicians and ancillary workers whose main aim is to improve the standards of care of the cancer patient. Remember that:

> Cancer is a potentially treatable disease.
> Always stage and check the diagnosis.
> Never stop evaluating treatment.
> Communication should take place at all levels.
> Every symptom is not sinister.
> Rehabilitation and terminal care are active processes.

With these principles in mind it is now possible to consider the treatment available for the patient with cancer.

Part 3

The Treatment of Cancer

12 The Surgical Treatment of Cancer

For many years surgery was the only form of treatment available to the patient with cancer. As surgical techniques improved, together with intensive care support, it became surgically possible to attack tumours located in almost any site of the body. Surgery remains one of the most useful methods of cancer treatment and its role has now expanded to include reconstruction, diagnostic procedures and staging.

REMOVAL OF THE PRIMARY TUMOUR

This remains the role, par excellence, of surgery. The primary tumour, no matter where it is located, is removed, and the adjacent or contiguous organs resected. There is often the problem of knowing whether or not the tumour has been completely excised. In this case repeated biopsies and 'frozen sections' should be performed at the time of operation. Removal of the primary tumour as an aim of treatment assumes that this is possible without prejudicing the life of the patient. It also assumes that the patient has presented early enough for this to be carried out. It should be emphasised that if the primary tumour is small and has remained localised then surgery alone may be curative.

OPERATIVE TECHNIQUES

There is no place in this book to discuss operative methods in detail but the following paragraphs outline the principles involved.

Adequate Pre-operative Preparation

This essential preparation implies attention not only to biochemical, nutritional and haematological aspects of the case, but to the preparation of the patient himself, including a discussion with the patient of the operation to be carried out, the side effects of that operation and the construction of any unusual anatomical features, such as a colostomy. In head and neck operations difficulties with speech or the formation of a tracheostomy should be discussed with the patient.

Planning the Incision: the Approach to the Tumour

It has been repeatedly demonstrated that handling of a malignant tumour releases into the circulation showers of malignant cells. Although it has not been conclusively shown that this significantly increases the incidence of metastatic disease it is an important principle that the tumour should be handled as little as possible. Wherever it is feasible the blood supply to the tumour should be divided before mobilisation. Thus in the removal of colonic tumours ligation of blood supply before resection is said to improve survival rates. Carcinomas of the kidney may be removed either through a loin incision, or by an anterior approach, the latter enabling ligation of the renal vessels prior to removal and allowing less handling of the tumour.

En-bloc Excision of the Cancer

Most operative procedures are designed to remove the primary tumour in its entirety, together with adjacent lymph nodes. With carcinoma of the stomach, a partial gastrectomy would include not only removal of part of the stomach but the lesser omentum and lymph nodes, the greater omentum and perhaps the spleen, the whole specimen being removed intact. Similarly in a carcinoma of tongue with neck node involvement the specimen would include the tongue, neck nodes excised as a 'block dissection', together with part of the mandible.

Adequate Excision of the tumour

It is essential that an adequate margin of surrounding normal tissue is removed in order to be sure that the neoplasm has been completely excised. In carcinoma of the lung where a lobectomy is carried out it is imperative that the line of excision is at least 3 cm from the primary tumour. With cutaneous melanomas an area of skin at least 5 cm in radius from the tumour edge must be excised if satellite tumours are to be effectively removed, and this means that skin grafting is necessary in almost all instances and that primary closure is almost never adequate. However, for technical reasons, it may be impossible to be absolutely certain that the tumour has been adequately excised. It is important to review the pathological report and to consider further therapy where excision has not been complete.

Exploration Following Excision

In addition to obtaining a biopsy from the primary tumour and excising it, it is essential to carry out a complete exploration of the area under investigation and to perform any other procedures required. Thus, during a laparotomy for a carcinoma of pancreas, suspiciously enlarged lymph nodes should be biopsied and any hepatic metastases noted. At the time of laparotomy radio-opaque markers should be positioned in case subsequent radiotherapy is required. Localisation of the tumour site is thus improved. Bone marrow biopsy or biopsy of suspected tumour deposits outside the operative field, e.g. enlarged lymph nodes should be performed as indicated.

REMOVAL OF THE REGIONAL LYMPH NODES

There is considerable debate as to the advantages and disadvantages of removal of regional lymph nodes. Many of the arguments are based on the results of animal experiments which cannot be directly applied to the human situation. However, clinical trials with specific tumours should, in the near future, give an answer to this question. On the one hand there is some evidence that the regional nodes possess important regulatory functions at an immunological level. Removal of the nodes may therefore be positively harmful. In the meantime it is reasonable to conclude that obviously involved nodes should be removed but that nodes clinically not involved be left. There are important exceptions to this, notably when the presence or absence of tumour in lymph nodes may affect the staging of the patient and hence may affect the decision to combine surgery with other forms of therapy.

PALLIATIVE SURGICAL PROCEDURES

In the previous discussions it has been assumed that the tumour could be completely excised with no obvious metastases being noted. This may be described as curative surgery. On the other hand, patients may present with neoplasms which cannot be completely excised or are associated with spread outside the primary site. In this situation a different approach is usually adopted.

Carcinoma of the stomach is a good example of the problems which may arise, as many patients still present with lesions which are essentially inoperable. Faced with a bulky tumour or with peritoneal spread the surgeon has several alternatives, outlined below.

(1) He may decide to do nothing and close the abdomen, either because there would be great technical difficulties in resecting the tumour or because the widespread nature of the disease makes the prognosis seem hopeless.

(2) He may decide that symptomatic control is necessary and therefore a by-pass operation is performed. This would prevent vomiting.

(3) It may be possible to remove the bulk of the tumour, knowing that some will be left behind. This may be carried out even in the presence of obvious liver or peritoneal metastases. Such a procedure cannot be considered curative but may allow the more effective use of other forms of therapy.

Thus, using the example of carcinoma of the stomach, anything from nil to a complete resection may be performed, depending on the appearance of the tumour at laparotomy. These varied approaches pose several questions.

(1) What is the value of removing as much tumour as is technically feasible, assuming that this can be performed without greatly increasing the risks to the patient, knowing that some tumour has been left behind? The main value in removing tumour is that it makes subsequent radiotherapy or

chemotherapy more likely to be successful because of bulk tumour removal.

(2) What range of palliative procedures is available? In the gastrointestinal tract, numerous methods have been devised usually involving a resection or a by-pass operation. In the oesophagus a range of tubes is available which, if successfully inserted, allow swallowing to occur without obstruction. In a similar manner, obstruction of the urinary outflow can be by-passed.

(3) What is the value of local toilet in palliative treatment? There is no doubt that with a fungating lesion it is much more useful to try, wherever possible, to remove the lesion, even though residual tumour may be left behind. This is especially the case with breast carcinomas which may be extremely unpleasant for the patient.

(4) What is the role of surgery in the treatment of solitary metastases? In some instances, for example a secondary neoplasm involving the right lobe of the liver, it is perfectly justifiable to perform a partial hepatectomy. Similarly with a solitary lung or bone metastases local excision may offer a good chance of completely removing the lesion. This is said to be particularly the case in renal carcinomas.

(5) What is the role of emergency operative treatment in patients with advanced disease? This is an extremely difficult question to answer, though it is not an uncommon problem. Bleeding from the stomach or colon, intestinal obstruction and severe dyspnoea due to tracheal compression are exceptionally difficult to deal with and require judgement and technical expertise of a very high order. There are, in addition, complications of chemotherapy and radiotherapy which may also require operative intervention in a very ill patient. These include bleeding due to low platelet counts, infection related to immunosuppression, and intestinal obstruction related to radiation therapy. No simple advice can be given as to the management of such patients. The guiding principle must be to undertake procedures where an improvement of the quality of life of such patients can be expected.

THE ROLE OF SURGERY IN DIAGNOSIS, STAGING AND INVESTIGATION

Surgical methods are the most commonly used to make a definite diagnosis of cancer. Biopsy procedures are regularly performed and should be carried out with great care. It is essential to know beforehand whether or not special methods of examination of the tissue are to be required, e.g. electron microscopy, or whether special assays are to be carried out on the specimen, e.g. hormone assays or receptor assays in carcinoma of the breast.

In cases where the diagnosis of cancer is suspected the surgeon may be asked to perform a biopsy of an area known to be associated with spread. Thus a scalene node biopsy in a patient with a suspected carcinoma of lung may save a thoracotomy, or laparotomy may be the only way in which to settle the diagnostic issue. With increasing use of endoscopic methods including laparoscopy this need is becoming less, though it still remains of great value in the individual case.

In some cases, even when the diagnosis has been confirmed, the surgeon is called to carry out a staging procedure. This is particularly the case in certain lymphomas. The question posed on examination of the patient is: 'Is the disease confined to a single lymph node region or has it spread?' Prior to laparotomy the patient will require a full blood count, chest x-ray, lymphangiogram and, where possible, liver and spleen scintiscan. A bone marrow examination is also essential and, if infiltrated, precludes the need for laparotomy. At laparotomy the spleen is removed for full histological examination, and biopsies are performed of the lobes of the liver and any enlarged lymph nodes or those previously noted to be involved. The ovaries may be fixed behind the uterus to try to prevent their irradiation, should this be necessary. As described in a previous section this approach, aggressive as it may seem, does allow a much more logical approach to tumour treatment. In some forms of leukaemia it may be necessary, for therapeutic reasons, to perform splenectomy.

RECONSTRUCTIVE SURGERY

Surgical methods are often of great value in the rehabilitation of the patient following a mutilating operation. The use of standard plastic surgical techniques of skin grafting or the creation of flaps or pedicles may greatly improve the patient's outlook on life.

HORMONAL ABLATIVE PROCEDURES

Some cancers, notably those of the breast, prostate and uterus may be hormone dependent (chapter 7). Various operations have been used to manipulate hormone levels and these include oophorectomy, adrenalectomy and hypophysectomy. Following such operations replacement therapy may be necessary. Some tumours of endocrine glands themselves may be responsible for the secretion of excess hormone, also, as mentioned earlier, other neoplasms such as carcinomas of the lung secrete ectopic hormones. The complete removal of such tumours results in the disappearance of the abnormalities related to the hormones released.

COMPLICATIONS OF SURGICAL TREATMENT

Patients having surgical treatment for cancer have the same forms of postoperative morbidity as other patients having other types of operations. Such complications may be important as they may affect the use, and timing, of other forms of treatment. Thus a wound infection in a mastectomy scar would prevent the use of post-operative radiotherapy. The presence of a pelvic collection of pus would delay the use of chemotherapy. Patients with cancer tend to have a higher incidence of post-operative deep venous thrombosis and it may be of value to use some form of prophylaxis against this problem.

There are, however, some very specific forms of complications relating to cancer surgery. Some of these are closely associated with the mutilating effect of surgery including amputations and disfiguring facial or head and neck operations, and hence the value of pre-operative preparation of the patient. For example, mastectomy is psychologically a very traumatic event and careful post-operative handling by individuals skilled in this aspect of patient care is required. With colostomies or ileostomies, sound advice is also invaluable. Operations on the larynx or tongue where speech difficulties are anticipated also require careful pre- and post-operative management.

13 Radiotherapy

The use of radiation in the treatment of cancer began around the turn of the century when it became established that radiation had a very potent therapeutic effect on superficial cancers. Since that time there have been numerous advances in the use of radiation and now most forms of cancer may be treated by one or other types of ionising radiation. Radiotherapy, therefore, is an extremely valuable therapeutic weapon against cancer. Its prime value lies in the fact that, under appropriate conditions, it is an excellent method for locally controlling tumour growth. In this respect it is similar to surgery, and is subject to the same limitations, e.g. the volume which can be treated will depend on the extent of the disease, and the effect on normal surrounding tissues must be borne in mind. Like surgery, radiotherapy has no direct effect on secondary tumours outside the treated area.

THE BIOLOGICAL EFFECTS OF RADIATION

Radiation may be delivered to the body in a variety of ways, with a range of different machinery and equipment which will be described later. In general the effects of radiation at a cellular level are essentially the same no matter how it is applied to the patient.

Radiation may kill cells directly by acting at the level of DNA (chapter 4, p. 41). It may also prevent cells dividing and hence inhibit growth. Although some cells may not be killed directly they may die earlier than usual because of sub-lethal damage. If it were as simple as this then radiotherapy, if given in the correct dose, would invariably kill tumour cells and result in tumour regression. Several factors, however, make the situation less than ideal.

Damage to Normal Tissues

If high doses of radiation are used then not only cancer cells but normal cells die. As cancer cells are less efficient in repairing damage than normal cells it is hoped that, given the correct timing of treatment, normal cells will recover faster than cancer cells (figure 13.1) and their function be maintained. This emphasises, however, that radiation is not selective and that damage to normal tissues may be a limiting factor.

Radioresponsiveness of Tumours

While it is true that all cancer cells, and all normal cells, can be killed by the use of radiotherapy, in practice it is clear that some tumour types are more

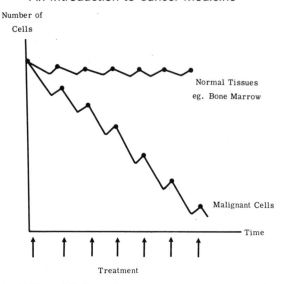

Figure 13.1   Differential effect of treatment on normal and malignant cells

sensitive to radiotherapy than others. This has led to the use of the terms 'radiosensitive' and 'radioresistant'. These terms should be abandoned as all tumours may be sensitive if given the correct dosage. In clinical terms it is well recognised that some forms of cancer, e.g. lymphomas, sarcomas, carcinomas, will respond well to radiotherapy, whilst others, e.g. adenocarcinoma of the gastrointestinal tract, respond less well.

Anatomical and Pathological Variations in Tumours

It is recognised that solid tumours are not composed of homogenous masses of identical tumour cells. They are a mixture of tumour cells and stromal cells; they contain blood vessels and the nutrition of sections of the tumour may be poor and there may be areas of necrosis. Radiation therapy is less effective in areas of hypoxia and the blood supply of the tumour, and the amount and character of the stroma may affect the responsiveness. These effects may be partially overcome by the use of hyperbaric oxygen to decrease the hypoxia or by the use of radiosensitisers.

Cell Survival and Cell Kinetic Data

Within any individual tumour it is known that only a proportion of the cells will be in division, the growth fraction (figure 13.2). Radiation therapy will kill cells in the growth fraction preferentially but this leaves a proportion of cells dormant. These cells may become capable of dividing (clonogenic cells) and it is therefore essential that the course of radiotherapy is given over a sufficient

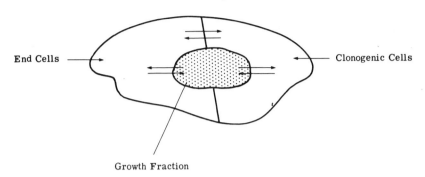

Figure 13.2   Tumour kinetics – a diagrammatic illustration of the compartmentalisation of a tumour into growing and non-growing fractions

period of time to cover this eventuality. As it is often not clear how many viable cells remain following therapy, recurrence of the tumour may follow.

The above points have been made in order that the fractionation schedules and dosages of radiotherapy are more clearly understood. They also illustrate some of the reasons for recurrence of tumour in a previously irradiated area. Some of these criticisms apply in a similar way to the use of chemotherapy.

METHODS OF ADMINISTERING RADIATION THERAPY

There are two main methods of administering radiotherapy. The first is to use radioactive isotopes which disintegrate, releasing particles of varying types. The second is the use of electrical methods to produce radiation artificially. These x-ray machines are of several types, each designed to produce radiation of different energies. These energies are related to the potential difference applied at the x-ray source and this is how machines are classified. The higher the voltage the greater the penetration of the x-rays. A radioactive source is used to emit gamma rays.

X-ray Machines

Superficial voltage (10–140 kilovolt). These machines produce x-rays, with limited penetration. They are used for the treatment of skin cancers.

Deep x-ray therapy units (250 kilovolt). Orthovoltage units. Because of the increased penetration resulting from the potential difference employed, these machines can be used to treat tumours in most areas of the body. Some years ago they were the standard units available in most Radiotherapy departments.

Megavoltage or supervoltage units. These produce x-rays, from sources of 4–8 megavolts. The most usual machine is the Linear accelerator. In this machine, electrons are accelerated in a straight line along an evacuated tube. The Betatron is another machine which causes electrons to travel in a circular path, moving with increasing energy. Up to 20 megavolt can be produced in this way. These machines can now be used to treat almost all forms of cancer except for superficial tumours.

Gamma ray beam units. This consists of a heavily shielded radioactive source with an aperture through which the x-rays emerge. The normal sources of gamma rays are cobalt 60 (the cobalt bomb unit) or caesium 137. These methods are sometimes referred to as telecurie therapy.

Particle Therapy

A variety of ionising particles may be used in the treatment of cancer. Alpha particles are little used nowadays. Newer developments include the use of pi-mesons, though a much greater amount of research is required before any comment can be made of their usefulness. The particles in common use are as follows:

(1) Beta rays. These consist of electrons, and have a limited power of penetration. They may be used in the following forms of therapy. (a) Surface therapy in the treatment of skin lesions. An applicator of Strontium 90 may be used. (b) Intracavity therapy. The injection of radioisotopes into pleural or ascitic fluids has been used to control effusions. Radioactive gold and phosphorus have been employed. (c) Systemic therapy with radioiodine in thyroid cancer and thyrotoxicosis, and radiophosphorus in polycythaemia have an important part to play in the management of these conditions.

(2) Neutrons. Equipment capable of producing neutrons has recently become available. Neutron therapy has a potential advantage in neoplasms in which oxygen deficiency occurs. Currently the machines are being evaluated and initially promising results reported.

The Use of Seeds, Needles and Tubes

Radioactivity may be packaged in a variety of ways using radium or one of its substitutes. When placed inside needles these can then be inserted close to the neoplasm so that the maximum effect can be obtained. Radon, a radioactive gas, with a very short half-life is also used in the form of seeds, usually introduced by a special 'gun'. In certain forms of gynaecological cancer, e.g. cancer of the cervix, intracavitary (intrauterine) insertion of radium inside a tube and ovoid radium applicators are used in the vault of the vagina.

PRINCIPLES OF TREATMENT AND DOSAGES

Radioactivity can be measured in several ways, the most important clinical unit being the rad. The rad measures not the energy released by the source, but the actual amount absorbed by the tissues. One rad is equivalent to 100 ergs/gram. By knowing the amount of radioactivity on the surface of the body (measured in roentgens) and by knowing the absorptive properties of the tissue, it is possible to calculate the number of rads absorbed by the organs. The absorptive properties vary from tissue to tissue.

When external radiation is used to treat a patient with an internal cancer it is possible to calculate the dosage in rads which will be delivered to the tissue. These isodose curves (figure 13.3) are essential in planning treatment. There is a major difference depending on whether megavoltage or superficial x-ray therapy is used. By using megavoltage therapy there is improved dosage deeper in the tissues. It is also possible to have better beam definition and the side effects related to skin lesions or bone necrosis are less.

When individual tumours are considered for treatment by external irradiation it is necessary to know the isodose curves for the particular machine used. If carcinoma of the oesophagus is taken as an example (figure 13.4) it can be seen that with a single field the dosage achieved may be inadequate. Using parallel pairs the dosage to the tumour is increased, and by the use of parallel opposed pairs of fields the tumour is given an even more effective dosage. By calculation, it is possible to provide the radiotherapist with the data which will allow the most appropriate use of the facilities available. Computer simulation units now make this task more efficient and reliable.

Before treatment is instituted the tumour is localised as best as possible radiologically, the skin tattooed or a mould made in order that the treatment is given to the same area each time. Where the tumour is superficial lead wedges are used to shield the skin area. When important internal organs are not involved in the neoplastic process, shielding is also used.

The actual amount of radiation given to an individual patient depends on the dosage required to eradicate the cancer cells, and the time interval between each treatment. The dosage and time of treatment (fractionation) are interdependent. For superficial tumours a single dose may be sufficient. For deeper and larger lesions multiple doses will be required. The fractionation also allows recovery of normal tissue between doses. Thus for post-operative treatment of skin flaps, axilla and supraclavicular regions following mastectomy, 4000–4500 rads would be given over a period of 3–4 weeks. For localised bone lesions a five-day course delivering of 2000 rads might be used. For carcinoma of the larynx a parallel pair of fields delivering 6000 rads over five weeks might be employed. The dosage and timing will vary with the individual tumour and the individual patient.

THE USE OF RADIOTHERAPY IN THE TREATMENT OF CANCER

Radiotherapy is now used, almost exclusively, in the treatment of cancer. The particular value of external irradiation is the ability to localise therapy and so

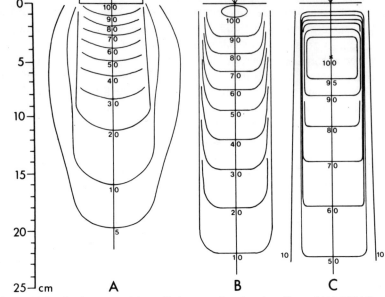

Figure 13.3   Isodose curves in radiotherapy showing the effect of (A) 200 kilovolts, (B) 2 megavolts, (C) 20 megavolts on the penetration of the radiation. The highest dose is labelled 100 per cent and other doses are expressed as a percentage of this. (Walter, J., *Cancer and Radiotherapy*, Churchill Livingstone, London, 1973)

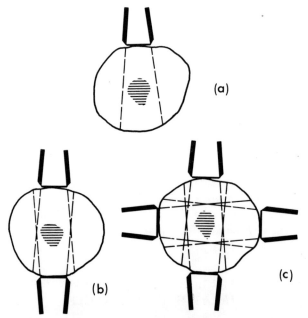

Figure 13.4   Comparison of three methods of approaching a tumour by radiotherapy: (a) single field, (b) parallel pair fields, (c) two pairs of opposed fields. (Walter, J., *Cancer and Chemotherapy*, Churchill Livingstone, London, 1973)

allow eradication of the tumour. It is thus used in the same way as surgery. Occasionally external radiation is used to treat the whole body, but this is worthwhile in only a limited range of cancers. The systemic use of radioactive isotopes in the treatment of widespread disease has likewise a very limited role.

Radiotherapy can be given prophylactically in certain instances. In this way it is used to eradicate small numbers of tumour cells either following surgery or to an area known to be associated with a high recurrence rate. Thus it is used to treat the area before overt disease is detectable. Following mastectomy for carcinoma of the breast the skin flaps may be irradiated to prevent local recurrence. In some of the sarcomas where there is known to be a high incidence of lung metastases, whole lung irradiation has been used to prevent their development. There are, however, problems associated with this.

The treatment of cancer by radiotherapy can be considered to be curative or palliative. In using radiation in a curative way it is essential that the disease is localised and the maximum amount of radiation given to the area without significantly affecting surrounding tissues and organs. Such radical radiotherapy, as it is usually called, requires considerable attention to detail and very careful planning. Curative radiotherapy is now used in a variety of neoplasms: the reticuloses, seminoma of the testes and neuroblastomas all respond well. When the disease is localised then radical radiotherapy may be used in the treatment of squamous carcinomas of the skin or head and neck. Some neoplasms, however, are known not to be so responsive to treatment, and the ability to eradicate cancer cells completely cannot be guaranteed. These include the adenocarcinomas of the gastrointestinal tract, carcinoma of the kidney, and malignant melanoma.

Palliative radiotherapy is used in a different way. It is assumed in this case that the primary tumour cannot be fully treated because of extent of disease or because the tumour has already spread. In this instance the aims of the therapy are different. They are now to control local tumour growth, to alleviate symptoms or to be used in conjunction with other forms of treatment such as chemotherapy. Palliative radiotherapy has an important part to play in the treatment of metastatic disease. Symptom relief and control of the neoplasm may be obtained.

Radiotherapy may be given on its own, or post-operatively. More recently, however, its use has been integrated with other forms of cancer therapy, and pre-operative radiotherapy now has an important part to play in the management of some tumours. Radiotherapy and chemotherapy are being increasingly used together.

Complications of Radiotherapy

Because of the known biological effects of radiation it is perhaps not surprising that its use is associated with side effects. With increasing sophistication of methodology and the availability of higher energy radiation, these side effects are diminishing. However, as the radiation usually penetrates normal tissues these will be involved to a greater or lesser extent. The complications may be divided into local or systemic.

The most important of the local complications is the effect on the skin. Radiation affects the skin in a variety of ways. Following the start of treatment there is a latent period which, depending on dosage and timing, is followed by the radiation reaction. Initially there is erythema associated with recoverable epilation. The redness may then increase and may be associated with pigmentation of the area and some peeling of the skin (dry desquamation). If further radiotherapy is given the surface may blister forming superficial ulcers (moist desquamation). At this stage loss of hair and sweat glands is permanent. During normal treatments none or all of the above may be noted. If treatment is continued ulceration may occur (radionecrosis) which is very slow to heal and may be extremely troublesome. It should be emphasised that with careful treatment planning this complication should be avoided. As the skin reaction dies down the area may be left completely normal or with pigmentation, atrophy and telangiectasia. It was noted in the early days of treatment that overdosage of the area could lead to the development of malignant change. This is almost never seen nowadays.

The skin reactions noted above are readily treated. The first essential is that the patient is informed that changes may occur. Thereafter the skin should be kept dry and not washed until the reaction has settled down. When superficial ulceration develops this may be treated topically with a variety of creams. Traditionally gentian violet has been used.

Radiation to mucous membranes may also produce serious side effects. Dryness of the mouth and pharynx following radiation to the area may be difficult to control. More frequently there are acute reactions with mouth ulceration, and if the gastrointestinal tract has been irradiated, diarrhoea with mucosal ulceration may occur. These effects occur acutely, and may be followed months or years later by fibrosis or stenosis. For example, radiation to the breast area may be followed by lung fibrosis, and pelvic irradiation for gynaecological malignancy may be associated with the development, in a small percentage of cases, of strictures of small or large bowel.

Unless superficial radiation is being used it is likely that bone will be irradiated during the course of treatment of internal cancer. The bone marrow is very sensitive to radiotherapy and, not surprising, haematological complications may occur. The total white blood count and the platelet count are reduced when a substantial proportion of active bone marrow is radiated. Such treatments also affect the immune response and the total lymphocyte count and various *in vitro* parameters of the immune response may be depressed for up to one year after therapy. Overdosage of osseous tissue may lead to bone necrosis.

When the gonads are irradiated even with low doses, significant effects may occur. Hormone release by the ovary or testis is abolished and, indeed, a radiation oophorectomy is used in the treatment of breast cancers.

Reproductive function is abolished though it may be recoverable. The possibility of chromosomal damage should be remembered.

Because radiotherapy may be associated with altering the DNA of the cell there is the possibility of an increase in the incidence of second malignancies. This also applies to the use of chemotherapy.

Other organs may be damaged during radiotherapy. They include the lens of the eye with the development of cataract, and the tear duct with blockage due to fibrosis. The kidney is usually shielded during treatment to prevent the development of radiation nephritis. Although, in general, nervous tissue is generally radioresistant, high doses will affect function. This is particularly the case with the spinal cord in which high doses may lead to paraplegia.

The systemic effects of radiotherapy include the haematological changes previously described. In addition, when deep x-ray therapy is used, radiation sickness may develop. The occurrence of this syndrome depends on the site of radiation and the volume treated. The syndrome is associated with tiredness, weakness, headache and nausea. There is no specific treatment at present but anti-emetics and the use of vitamin preparations have been advocated.

Cancer of the Breast

Radiotherapeutic techniques are used extensively in patients with breast cancer. As a modality of therapy it is used not only to treat primary site, but to treat metastatic disease especially in bone, and as a method of ablating ovarian function by direct irradiation of the ovaries.

Following mastectomy, the supraclavicular, axillary and parasternal nodes may be irradiated (figure 13.5). The chest wall may be irradiated either at the

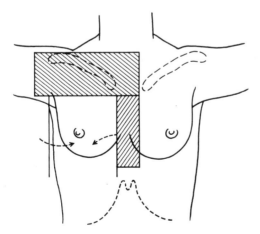

Figure 13.5   Radiotherapeutic fields used to treat patient's post-mastectomy. The internal mammary lymph nodes, supraclavicular nodes and axillary nodes are irradiated. (Robinson, *Surgery*, Longman, London)

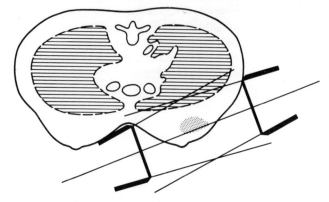

Figure 13.6   Diagram to show the use of a tangential field to treat the chest wall in patients with breast cancer. There is minimal radiation dosage to the lungs. (Walter, J., *Cancer and Radiotherapy*, Churchill Livingstone, London, 1973)

site of a mastectomy scar in an attempt at eliminating all viable tumour cells, or in the presence of the primary breast cancer (figure 13.6). Tangential fields are used, minimising damage to lung tissue. These methods illustrate the use of external beam therapy.

Cancer of the Body of Uterus

A knowledge of the extent of spread of uterine cancer dictates the kind of therapy to be used. Intracavity radium is inserted, the amount of radium being accurately calculated. It is subsequently removed at a specified time interval based on the dose of radiation to be given (figure 13.7). It is usual to

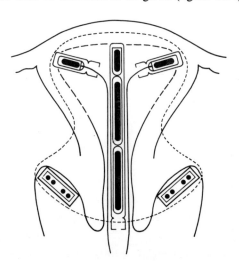

Figure 13.7   Use of intracavity irradiation in carcinoma of the uterus. Ovoids containing radioactive material are placed in the vaginal fornices. (Marie Curie Hospital)

pack the lateral fornices of the vagina with radium to deal with spread into the cervix and vagina. This demonstrates the use of intracavity irradiation using radium sources and emphasises the importance of careful calculation of the dose to be given and removal at specific times following insertion.

Carcinoma of the Tongue or Floor of Mouth

In appropriate lesions radiotherapeutic techniques may be used to treat such tumours. External beam therapy is used in most cases. In some, however, radium needle implants may be used (figure 13.8). Under general anaesthesia

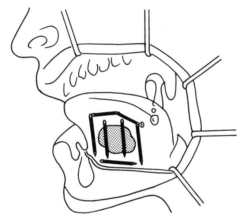

Figure 13.8   Use of radioactive needles in the treatment of carcinoma of the tongue. The needles are left in place for a fixed length of time and then removed. (Paterson, C. R., *Treatment of Malignant Disease*, Edward Arnold, London)

special applicators are used to insert the needles in a manner calculated to give the correct dosage to the neoplasm. Each needle is attached to a silk thread which is used to remove them when the computed dose has been given. Such techniques are less readily used now than previously. However, the use of needle implants in various sites of the body may be a very valuable adjunct to therapy.

Hodgkin's Disease

This tumour is particularly responsive to radiotherapy. The treatment of this particular neoplasm highlights the importance of staging and treatment planning. When the disease is confined to lymph nodes above the diaphragm radiotherapy to the 'mantle' area may be given (figure 13.9). The treatment area covers lymph node areas in the upper part of the body. When the disease involves only the lymph nodes below the diaphragm an inverted-Y radiation field is used (figure 13.9). When both areas are involved but the disease is confined to lymph nodes both techniques are employed.

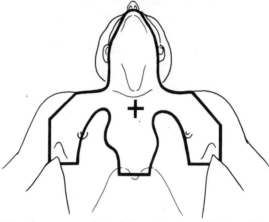

Figure 13.9   Use of upper mantle technique for the radiation of lymph node areas above the diaphragm. Note the extension of the field into the mediastinum, axillae and neck

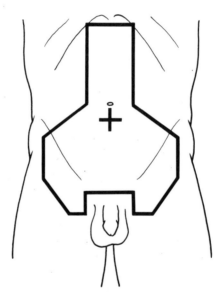

Figure 13.10   Use of the inverted-Y technique for the irradiation of lymph node areas below the diaphragm

Other Forms of Cancer

The few examples chosen above illustrate some of the many radiotherapeutic techniques which are currently in use. Many others are employed in other sites. They are all, however, based on careful planning of treatment, avoidance or shielding of important normal organs, and correct calculation of dosage and timing (fractionation) of therapy.

14 Cancer Chemotherapy

Compared to radiotherapy and surgery, chemotherapy is a relatively new modality of treatment for cancer. When chemotherapeutic agents, including antibiotics, became widespread in the treatment of bacterial infections, it was natural that a search would be made for a 'magic bullet' which would selectively kill all cancer cells. The search still continues for the ideal drug though, in the meantime, over 30 active drugs have been discovered and are in regular clinical use (figure 14.1). It is no exaggeration to say that the development of effective drugs to treat cancer has significantly modified the clinical course of various types of cancers and, perhaps even more so, has altered the philosophy of treatment for many tumours.

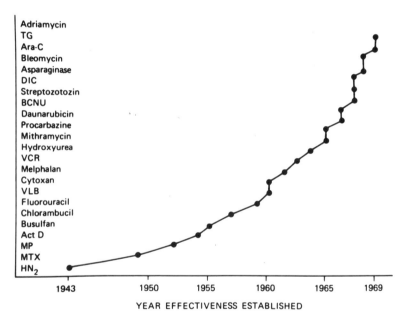

Figure 14.1 Availability of clinically effective chemotherapeutic agents over the past thirty years illustrating the increasing number of drugs which have recently become available

DRUG DEVELOPMENT AND SCREENING

The earlier chemotherapeutic agents were discovered by serendipity or by the application of biochemical principles to design new drugs which would inhibit specific metabolic pathways or to modify existing drugs. While these processes continue, in addition, large programmes have been instituted to discover new and better agents, starting from two points. (1) A compound is discovered or developed which is considered to be effective against tumours *in vivo*. (2) A series of compounds with no known activity but which are potentially useful are screened against a variety of tumours in animals.

At the conclusion of these studies a compound may be identified which is active against a range of cancers in small animals. This process may take a great deal of time and is extremely expensive. Having identified such a compound it is now appropriate to carry out clinical trials. These are usually carried out in three phases.

A phase 1 study of the drug is carried out to investigate its toxicity, its pharmacological effects, and its mode of administration. Such trials are usually performed on patients with advanced cancer. At the conclusion of this phase it should be possible to have sufficient information on the clinical pharmacology of the drug for it to be tested more rigorously.

In the phase 2 study the drug is given to groups of patients with specific tumours. The drug is given in the most appropriate dosage and route, and the object is to identify those tumours which are particularly responsive.

The phase 3 study is designed to investigate, in greater detail, drug effectiveness against tumours for a range of neoplasms. Differing dose schedules and routes of administration are tried and an estimate of responsiveness obtained.

At the conclusion of these studies sufficient information should be available on the drug in order that it can be used in appropriate dosages and in the most responsive tumours. It is a fact, however, that such single agent data is not yet available for all drugs, or for all tumours. Following the definition of a drug as being active as a single agent in a particular tumour it may then be used in combination with other drugs.

CLASSIFICATION OF CANCER CHEMOTHERAPEUTIC AGENTS

It is usual to classify drugs according to their site of action on the metabolic pathways of the cell. This has some merit but often oversimplifies the problem as each drug may have more than one site of action. In addition this method takes no account of action of the drug at various phases of the cell cycle. It is necessary, therefore, to classify the biological action of drugs in at least two ways: (1) in relation to the site of action, (2) in relation to their action in the cell cycle.

Alkylating Agents

These agents include nitrogen mustard, mitomycin C, myleran, the nitrosoureas, the triazenes, melphelan and cyclophosphamide. All of these compounds have in common one or more highly reactive alkyl groups which, under biological conditions, can transfer that group to a receptor. The receptor may be a protein but it is usually a nucleic acid, particularly DNA. The binding of the alkyl group inhibits DNA function and produces fragmentation and clumping of chromosomes. Bifunctional or polyfunctional agents are more effective because of their ability to cross-link strands of nucleic acid. The binding would appear to be predominantly to guanine residues. Many of the compounds noted above are inactive *in vitro*, and require metabolic activation to produce the effective compound. Cyclophosphamide is a particular example of this.

Antimetabolites

These compounds act by blocking the synthesis of essential metabolites, usually of DNA or RNA. They are normally enzyme inhibitors. The antimetabolites include methotrexate, the pyrimidine antagonists 5-fluorouracil and cytosine arabinoside, the purine antagonists azaserine, 6-thioguanine, 6-mercaptopurine and azothiopurine. Each of these compounds acts at different sites in the metabolic pathways leading to the synthesis of DNA or RNA.

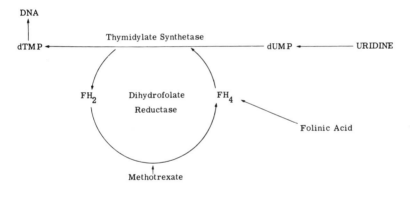

FH_2 = dihydrofolate FH_4 = Tetrahydrofolate

Figure 14.2   Mechanism of action of methotrexate on the enzyme thymidylate synthetase

Methotrexate, or amethopterin, is a good example of this (figure 14.2). It is a folic acid antagonist and acts by inhibiting dihydrofolate reductase, an essential enzyme in the transfer of an additional carbon in the synthesis of thymidine and its incorporation into DNA.

It is important to point out that methotrexate may act at other levels notably in the direct inhibition of the synthesis of thymidylate. It is also important to appreciate that the biochemical effects of methotrexate can be overcome by giving large doses of folinic acid. This information is of clinical relevance where very large doses of methotrexate are given (high dose methotrexate). Following administration, normal cells are 'rescued' by giving folinic acid.

5-Fluorouracil is structurally very similar to the natural compound uracil (figure 14.3).

It blocks not only RNA synthesis by inhibiting incorporation of uracil into RNA, but also DNA synthesis, by blocking the synthesis of thymidylate. The enzyme thymidylate synthetase is inhibited (figure 14.3).

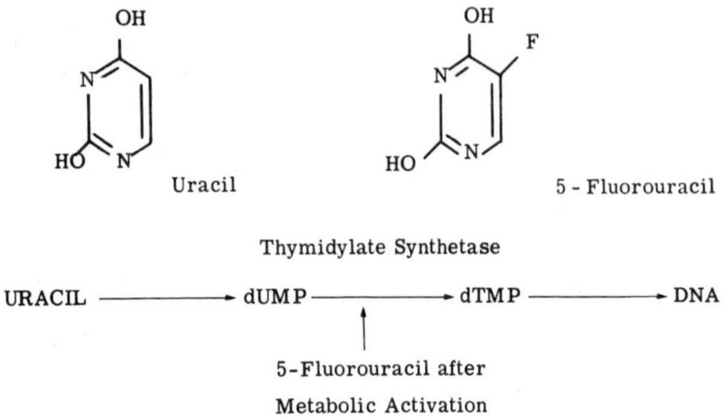

Figure 14.3   Comparison between uracil, the normal metabolite and 5-fluorouracil. After metabolism, the 5-fluorouracil acts by inhibiting DNA synthesis. Other mechanisms of actions are possible

Antibiotics

A wide range of antimitotic antibiotics have been used clinically. These include actinomycin, cycloheximide, mithramycin, streptonigrin, adriamycin, daunomycin, bleomycin, streptozotocin, and mitomycin C.

These compounds act in a variety of ways and their often complex chemical structure has frequently made it difficult to investigate this fully. Some, such as cycloheximide and puromycin, inhibit protein synthesis while others bind to DNA. It is well known, for example, that actinomycin D inhibits DNA-dependent RNA synthesis. The antibiotics show clearly how the molecular structure of the compound is related to activity. Adriamycin and daunomycin differ only in the presence or absence of a hydroxyl group. This substitution considerably alters the spectrum of activity of the two drugs, daunomycin being specially active in the leukaemias, and adriamycin in solid tumours.

Vinca Alkaloids

The two most important of these plant-derived alkaloids are vincristine and vinblastine. These two compounds have slightly different spectrums of clinical activity and side effects but both act by arresting cells in mitosis. Their mechanism of action as spindle poisons is still not clear.

Miscellaneous Agents

A number of active drugs cannot be classified as shown above, either because the mechanism of action is still not known, or because they have quite different sites of activity. Asparaginase, for example, was discovered when certain mouse neoplasms were found to be inhibited in the presence of guinea pig serum. The active factor was identified as the enzyme asparaginase and it was subsequently found that asparagine was an essential amino acid in some forms of leukaemia cells.

MECHANISM OF ACTION OF DRUGS IN RELATION TO THE CELL CYCLE

Although often difficult to define, dividing cells go through a series of phases between one mitosis and the next (pp. 20–22). It has been found experimentally that some drugs act preferentially on only one phase of the cell cycle (cycle specific) while others act at all stages (cycle non-specific). Most drugs have no effect if the cell is not in division (G_0). Using small animal models with corroborative evidence in humans it is possible to place most drugs into one of these two classes (table 14.1).

Table 14.1   Classification of drugs according to their action on the cell cycle

Cycle specific	Cycle non-specific
S phase: Cytosine arabinoside, hydroxyurea, methotrexate 5-fluorouracil	Cyclophosphamide Nitrosoureas Actinomycin D
Mitosis: Vinca alkaloids, bleomycin	Daunomycin

These differences may be of considerable importance in the design of combinations of chemotherapy.

RELATIONSHIP BETWEEN CHEMOTHERAPEUTIC AGENTS AND GROWTH KINETICS OF TUMOURS

Tumours consist essentially of three compartments, each closely interrelated (see figure 13.2).

(1) The proliferating compartment (growth fraction) containing cells in the process of division.

(2) The non-clonogenic compartment consisting of end cells or cells which have lost the capacity to divide.

(3) The clonogenic compartment comprising cells which, although not in division at the time, may divide if an appropriate stimulus is given.

Chemotherapeutic agents act mainly on the dividing fraction, and almost never on the clonogenic compartment. The non-proliferating compartment is of less interest, but may form a large part of the tumour. Thus the response obtained by a particular drug against a tumour depends a great deal on the size of the proliferating compartment. If the growth fraction is large then the potential for cell kill is greater. If it is small then there is less chance of an effective drug response.

The cytotoxic action of chemotherapeutic agents obeys first order kinetics, i.e. for a given dose of drug the same proportion of cells is killed on each occasion the drug is administered, and not the same number of cells. Figure 14.4 shows the effect of a hypothetically very active drug, when it kills cells in this way. Treatment is given at point A, and with a 99 per cent cell kill the cell number is reduced from 10^{12} to 10^{10}. At point C the same drug, producing the same 99 per cent cytotoxicity, reduces the cell number from 10^8 to 10^6. This is a marked difference in the number of cells killed though the proportion remains the same.

Under ideal circumstances (see figure 13.1) the number of tumour cells would be sequentially reduced until the tumour was eliminated. However, as normal cells, and in particular the bone marrow, may also be affected by the drug, this must also be taken into account. If the growth fraction of the tumour is larger than that of the marrow, then marrow recovery can take

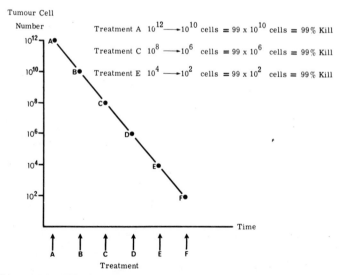

Figure 14.4   Effective drug therapy. Cell kill follows first order kinetics

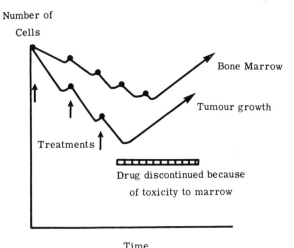

Figure 14.5   Effect of bone marrow toxicity on drug response. Tumour growth
occurs

place while the tumour volume is reducing in size (see figure 13.1). However, when the tumour has a small growth fraction, drug therapy may have to be stopped because of marrow toxicity. During this period of time the tumour continues to grow (figure 14.5). Although the tumour may be sensitive initially, resistance may develop and the tumour may 'escape' from drug effects and grow despite treatment (figure 14.6). An appreciation of tumour kinetics in relation to tumour size is also important when adjuvant chemotherapy is considered. This will be discussed later.

PREDICTIVE TEST OF ACTIVITY OF
CHEMOTHERAPEUTIC AGENTS

It would obviously be desirable if, before administration, the effectiveness of individual drugs could be tested against the patient's own tumour. This would be analagous to the plate testing of antibiotics used in bacterial chemotherapy. Although this has been attempted on many occasions either with organ cultures, cell cultures or tissue slices, the technical problems involved have not made it a feasible proposition at the present time. Research still continues and it is hoped that it will soon bear fruit.

PHARMACOLOGICAL ASPECTS OF CANCER CHEMOTHERAPY

In common with any other group of pharmacological agents, it is essential that the absorption, distribution, metabolism and excretion of these drugs are fully understood.

If absorption is considered then not only may patients with cancer show some evidence of malabsorption, but the drugs themselves may influence small bowel function. As many of the drugs require metabolic activation or deactivation by the liver, the presence or absence of liver metastases may significantly affect activity and toxicity. Cancer patients are not normal patients and it is unwise to assume that metabolic pathways will be the same as those in normal individuals. As the drugs may be nephrotoxic or be excreted in the urine adequate renal function is necessary.

In general terms, drugs can be considered to become compartmentalised on administration. They become distributed in blood where they may or may not be protein bound. There they exchange with other body fluids and become intracellular, affecting both normal cells and cancer cells. The pharmacological activity of the drugs depends a great deal on the proportion of drug which is actually taken up by the tumour itself. By a knowledge of the blood levels, excretion patterns and tumour uptake (the pharmacokinetics of the drug) it is possible to derive the most appropriate dose schedule for the individual patient. It is pertinent to point out that cancer patients may have pleural effusions or ascites. These fluid collections may act as a pharmacological 'third space' and sequester drug, so increasing toxicity because of accumulation and subsequent release into body fluids.

Drug dosages are usually calculated on a weight basis or in relation to surface area. The latter gives the most reproducible dosage schedules. When very large doses of drugs are to be used, or when the patient has had previous treatment with chemotherapy or radiotherapy, it may be worth using the principle of 'dose escalation', that is a smaller than calculated dose is used on the first occasion and, if there are no significant toxic effects, then on subsequent occasions the dose is increased to the desired level.

Drugs may be administered continuously or intermittently. Wherever possible it is usual to use intermittent schedules. Such schedules are associated with less short-term and long-term toxicity and some results have shown that intermittent administration has a superior anti-tumour effect.

Chemotherapeutic agents can be administered in a wide variety of ways. They may be given orally or intravenously. The intravenous route may include rapid injection or continuous infusion. Some drugs, e.g. Bleomycin or cytosine arabinoside may be given by intramuscular injection. A great deal of effort has been made to use drugs intra-arterially, by regional perfusion. In concept, this produces very high levels of drugs in the region of the neoplasm. Liver metastases and limb lesions have been studied using this method. In general the results compare with those obtained by intravenous injections. With some neoplasms there is good evidence that cells spread into the central nervous system. This is particularly the case with the acute leukaemias in which meningeal disease poses a special problem. As the drugs used may not penetrate the blood brain barrier they require to be given intrathecally. When pleural effusions or ascites are present drugs may be administered directly into the cavity. Finally drugs may be used topically. They may be given in various preparations to lesions on the skin, in the mouth or in the vagina. They may be instilled into the wound at the end of a surgical operation in an attempt at killing residual tumour cells. They may be instilled rectally or into the bladder to achieve high local concentrations of the drug.

MECHANISMS OF SELECTIVITY AND THE DEVELOPMENT OF RESISTANCE

The two major problems of cancer chemotherapy are to increase the selectivity of the drugs against tumours, and to prevent the development of resistance.

At the present time cytotoxic drugs affect both cancer cells and normal cells. There is little margin for error in that the maximum tolerated dose, (MTD) may be close to the minimum effective dose (MED). The ratio of MTD to MED, the therapeutic index, is often small, and dangerous consequences may occur from overdosage. Methods to increase the selectivity include the greater understanding of biochemical mechanisms in cancer cells and in the specific design of compounds which affect these processes. A second way to improve selectivity would be to utilise tissue-specific metabolic activation mechanisms, e.g. in liver or kidney, to localise drug therapy. Thirdly, by combining the drug with tumour-specific antibody it is possible that the drug would 'home' to the tumour cell. Other mechanisms, including the use of liposomes, will be discussed later.

The clinical problem of resistance to chemotherapeutic agents is important. It is frequently observed that a tumour will often respond rapidly, and to all intents completely, to drug therapy, only to recur. The tumour has become resistant to the drug and is able to grow freely in its presence (figure 14.6). The development of resistance is a complex phenomenon usually involving the development of an alternative metabolic pathway to by-pass the reaction

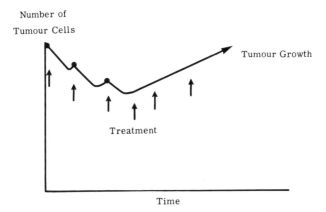

Figure 14.6   Effect of drug resistance on tumour growth. Following an initial response, the tumour develops resistance to the drug and growth occurs

inhibited by the drug. In the case of the alkylating agents, enzymes capable of excising and repairing damaged DNA are induced, and these agents then become ineffective (p. 41–2). Second line drugs may be used to achieve a second response if the alternative metabolic pathway is known.

SINGLE AGENT CHEMOTHERAPY

For many years it was considered best to administer drugs singly. The drug was given until a response was obtained and continued until the tumour recurred. This form of treatment produced valuable data on the use, toxicity and effectiveness of single drugs in specific tumour types. For several tumours this form of treatment is still applicable. It is also necessary to use drugs singly, during their development, to obtain enough information as to their usefulness in specific tumours.

COMBINATION CHEMOTHERAPY

More recently it has become common practice to use cytotoxic drugs in combinations, with two, three, four, five or six drugs being used simultaneously in the one patient. Combinations of drugs are used as their effectiveness has now been shown to be superior to the use of single drugs in many clinical situations. The principles governing the simultaneous use of several drugs are as follows.

(1) The drugs used should be active as single agents against the particular tumour type. This is stating the obvious, though it is not uncommon for drug combinations to include agents which are inactive against a specific tumour.

(2) Drugs having similar toxicity should be avoided.

(3) Drugs having different mechanisms of action, or different biochemical sites of action, should be used together.

(4) Drugs in combinations should be used as near as possible to their maximum doses when used as single agents. It is clearly of little benefit if drugs in combination can be only used at 20 per cent of their effective doses in order to prevent toxicity.

Although many of the drug combinations currently in use have been developed on the basis of clinical experience, increasing use is now being made of the knowledge of basic mechanisms of action of these drugs to inhibit metabolic pathways, and to act at specific times in the cell cycle.

Based on these principles various combinations of drugs have been devised to treat specific tumours. Combination chemotherapy has been very effective in increasing the response rates and length of response against many cancers. For Hodgkin's disease the complete remission rate using single agents is

25–30 per cent; with combination chemotherapy it becomes 70–80 per cent. In breast cancer the best that can be hoped for is a 20–30 per cent response rate with single drugs but up to 80 per cent response rates can be achieved with combinations. The same is true in many other cancers.

COMPLICATIONS OF CHEMOTHERAPY

Chemotherapy is associated with many side effects. When given in appropriate dosages and at the correct time intervals, these effects can be minimised. In many instances it is possible to use these drugs on an outpatient basis so allowing patients to go home or return to work.

Social Complications

Chemotherapy, given over a long period of time, necessitates repeated hospital visits or admissions. As such it may interrupt the routine life of the patient, and in some cases the patient has to travel long distances. In addition the non-specific complications of chemotherapy, as detailed below, may also interfere with normal life. In the elderly, drug administration may be a problem.

Non-specific Complications

These complications are common to most of the groups of drugs used, and includes the toxicity on the alimentary tract such as nausea, vomiting and diarrhoea. Such side effects may be overcome by the regular administration of the anti-emetics. Metabolic complications which occur include weight loss, anorexia and hypericaemia. When the latter is anticipated it is usual to start the patient on allopurinol. A number of dermatological problems have been reported including alopecia, skin pigmentation and nail changes. When some of the drugs used are extravasated from a vein into surrounding tissues, they are extremely irritant and local inflammation or tissue necrosis may occur. It is essential that great care is taken when these drugs are used.

During the course of chemotherapeutic drugs it is not unusual for gametogenesis to cease. Depending on the type of regimen used, up to 50 per cent of premenopausal women will cease to menstruate and they should be warned about this. Likewise in males spermatogenesis may be inhibited. The evidence, at present, suggests that this, *per se*, is not associated with subsequent abnormalities of the children of such patients if conception occurs. In the young male patient with a testicular tumour, it is worth considering sperm storage prior to chemotherapy.

Drug-specific Complications

In addition to the general problems listed above, most of the drugs used are associated with specific problems. These include:

Adriamycin	Alopecia, cardiotoxicity
Bleomycin	Pulmonary fibrosis, oral ulceration
Cyclophosphamide	Haemorrhagic cystitis
Methotrexate	Liver toxicity, oral ulceration
Vinca alkaloids	Neurotoxicity

Attention to proper dose scheduling, and limitation of amount of drug used, may prevent these occurring in some instances.

Haematological Toxicity

One of the most important consequences of the use of chemotherapy is the effect on the bone marrow. All elements of the marrow may be reduced with the attendant problems of bleeding (low platelets) or infection (leucopenia). Consequently these patients may require full supportive therapy (p. 97). Careful attention to dosage, route of administration and timing of treatment can minimise these problems.

Risk of Second Malignancy

One of the most worrying of all the complications is the risk of developing a second malignancy. This complication, though rare, is not entirely theoretical. In Hodgkin's disease and myeloma the long-term use of chemotherapy has been associated with an increased incidence of second neoplasms, notably the leukaemias. This increased risk may be related to chromosome changes caused by the drugs, to immunosuppression or to the activation of latent viruses. It may also be the case that patients who have developed one tumour are more likely to develop a second cancer.

THE DESIGN OF COMBINATION CHEMOTHERAPY FOR CLINICAL USE

It is often considered to be a matter of chance as to which drugs are used in a particular neoplasm. While this may have been the case several years ago, there should be no excuse at the present time for the indiscriminate or haphazard use of drugs. For most forms of cancer nowadays the drugs which are active against specific tumour are known. Even more importantly, drugs which are inactive or not even evaluated properly have been defined. Lists have been produced (table 14.2) which allow to be seen, at a glance, the number of drugs which are active, and those which are not. Drugs may be

Table 14.2   Cytotoxic drug evaluation in cancer patients

	Colon	Lung	Breast	Bladder	Sarcoma
++	5	5	7	2	4
+	2	6	7	0	2
−	19	14	10	0	0
NE	3	4	5	27	23

classified as being active (++), possibly active (+), inactive (−) or not evaluated (NE). Several points can be made.

(1) With cancer of the breast there are fourteen active drugs. It is possible therefore to design several combinations which, in theory, should be effective.

(2) If bladder cancer is considered, however, it can be seen that at the present time only two drugs are active and that to design combinations which include other drugs would be based on inadequate data: much more work is required with single agents in bladder cancer.

(3) Such tables are provisional and provide guidelines for the rational use of drugs and should not be used as a 'recipe book'.

With a number of active drugs against a particular tumour it becomes possible to design a combination for that tumour. It should be emphasised, however, that it is essential to check that the combination *is* better by carrying out the appropriate clinical trial. Drug combinations are selected on the basis of toxicities, mechanisms of action and known synergisms. A great deal of empiricism still remains at this stage of design. Evaluation, however, is the keynote. Some of the combinations which have been found to be effective in particular tumours are listed in table 14.3. It cannot be too strongly emphasised that the use of such combinations should be restricted to specific tumour sites.

Table 14.3   Drug combinations effective in particular tumours

Tumour	Drugs
Breast cancer	Cyclophosphamide, methotrexate and 5-fluorouracil, adriamycin, cyclophosphamide and vincristine
Colonic cancer	5-Fluorouracil and methyl CCNU
Hodgkin's disease	Nitrogen mustard, vincristine, procarbazine and prednisolone
Sarcomas	Adriamycin and cyclophosphamide, high dose methotrexate and vincristine
Myeloma	Melphelan and prednisolone
Lung cancer	Cyclophosphamide, methotrexate, CCNU, bleomycin

It must also be strongly emphasised that such combinations are given for illustration only. In a rapidly developing field they may soon be superseded or modified.

THE ROLE OF CHEMOTHERAPY IN THE TREATMENT OF CANCER

Drug therapy is being increasingly used in all forms of cancer. This is of particular relevance when combined modality therapy is considered since

Table 14.4

(a)

Cancers in which drugs have been responsible for some patients achieving a normal life span

Acute leukemia in children	Ewing's sarcoma
Hodgkin's disease	Wilm's tumour
Histiocytic lymphoma	Burkitt's lymphoma
Skin cancer	Retinoblastoma
Testicular carcinoma	Choriocarcinoma
Embryonal rhabdomyosarcoma	

(b)

Cancers in which responders to chemotherapy have had demonstrated improvement in survival

Ovarian carcinoma	Lymphocytic lymphomas
Breast carcinoma	Neuroblastoma
Adult acute leukaemias	Adrenal cortical carcinoma
Multiple myeloma	Malignant insulinoma
Endometrial carcinoma	Gastrointestinal cancer
Prostatic cancer	Osteogenic sarcomas

(c)

Cancers responsive to drugs for which clinically useful improvement in survival of responders has not been clearly demonstrated

Head and neck cancers	Oat cell carcinoma of the lung
Central nervous system cancer	Malignant carcinoid tumours
Endocrine gland tumours	Soft tissue sarcomas
Malignant melanoma	

(d)

Cancers only marginally responsive or unresponsive to chemotherapeutic agents

Hypernephroma	Pancreatic carcinoma
Bladder carcinoma	Hepatocellular carcinoma
Cancer of the oesophagus	Thyroid carcinoma
Epidermoid carcinoma of the lung	

---

chemotherapy is now an integral part of many management schemes. In table 14.4 tumours are grouped into (a) those in which survival has been significantly prolonged by the use of drugs, (b) those in which there is some evidence for this, and (c), (d) those in which no evidence is yet available to suggest that chemotherapy has contributed anything to the management. In solid tumours, chemotherapy may be used pre-operatively or post-operatively, and it may be used in advanced disease or when there is minimal tumour mass. It is the latter aspect which appears to hold greatest promise and will be discussed in a later section.

DRUG INTERACTION WITH NON-CYTOTOXIC AGENTS

Increasingly it is being recognised that in addition to there being interactions between cytotoxic drugs, there are also important relationships between chemotherapeutic agents and other drugs administered at the same time. The consequences of such interactions may be extremely serious and attention should always be paid to the drugs prescribed in any cancer patient. The following interactions are known to be significant and there may be many others still to be recorded.

(1) Methotrexate blood levels are altered by the administration of aspirin which affects the protein binding of the drug.

(2) Allopurinol inhibits the catabolism of 6-mercaptopurine and, if both drugs are to be used together, the dose of 6-mercaptopurine must be reduced.

(3) Cyclophosphamide metabolism may be altered by the simultaneous use of chlorpromazine.

(4) Anti-emetics and analgesics may alter gastric emptying and alter drug absorption.

(5) The non-absorbable antibiotics may also interfere with the absorption of chemotherapeutic agents.

15 Hormone Therapy in Cancer

As remarked earlier, the first endocrine procedure for the treatment of cancer was carried out in 1895 by Sir George Beatson. He performed oophorectomy in women with breast cancer and noted regression of metastatic deposits. The next advance came in 1941 when Huggins used oestrogens or orchidectomy to treat prostatic cancer. With the development of synthetic steroids it is not surprising that the role of hormones in the treatment of cancer has expanded considerably in recent years. Hormones are now used not only for treatment purposes but form an integral part of the overall management of the cancer patient. Recent advances in the understanding of the molecular role of hormones and the nature of receptors has encouraged a fresh look at hormones and cancer (see p. 74).

PREDICTION OF RESPONSE TO ENDOCRINE THERAPY

In patients with carcinoma of the breast approximately 30 per cent will respond to an alteration in the hormonal environment. As the treatment may involve the administration of hormones over a long period of time, or may require a surgical operation, it would be beneficial if methods were available to predict the response to endocrine therapy in individual patients. A great deal of investigative work has been done on urinary excretion products of steroid metabolism. Although the measurements obtained have provided methods of deciding which patients will, or will not, respond they are not sufficiently accurate. More recently the measurement of hormonal receptors, particularly oestrogen receptors in breast cancer tissue, has been employed. The breast tissue is removed, incubated with radioactive oestrogens and the amount of radioactivity taken up by the cytosol or the nucleus is estimated. Preliminary results have indicated that this may be a more sensitive method of predicting hormonal responsiveness.

CLINICAL USES OF HORMONE THERAPY

Carcinoma of Breast

This tumour is particularly responsive to endocrine therapy. The treatment used may either be with synthetic hormones, or with ablative operations which remove sources of hormone secretion. Patients with carcinoma of breast may be divided into pre-menopausal (including up to two years after the last menstrual period) and post-menopausal. The form of hormonal therapy varies depending on the menopausal status.

Pre-menopausal Patients

The main object is to remove the source of oestrogens, or to modify their effects by using androgens. Consequently oophorectomy, performed surgically or using radiotherapy, is an effective method of reduction of endogenous oestrogens. When a response occurs, it is usually rapid in onset, with a long duration. Up to 25 per cent of patients will respond to this procedure. When relapse occurs, following a good response, there is a good chance that a second response will be achieved by further reduction of endogenous oestrogens by adrenalectomy or hypophysectomy. The complications of such procedures in patients with advanced cancer should be taken into account before recommending their use.

An alternative form of treatment is to use androgenic steroids. Several are available commercially and may be given orally or intramuscularly. Response rates vary but are of the order of 20–30 per cent.

Post-menopausal Patients

Such patients have low endogenous oestrogen levels and tumour is often responsive to the administration of oestrogens. Traditionally, the synthetic oestrogen stilboestrol has been used at a dosage of 5 mg three times a day. More recently a new range of compounds has become available, the anti-oestrogens. These include Tamoxifen and Nafoxidine. Their mechanism of action is unclear at present but they may inhibit uptake of oestrogen by cytosol receptors. Adrenalectomy and hypophysectomy may also be used in post-menopausal patients.

There is some evidence that hormonal responsiveness increases with age, the over 70s being especially responsive to this form of therapy.

Male Breast Cancer

Although this is much rarer than female breast cancer, the evidence suggests that this, too, is a hormone responsive tumour. Small series have been reported suggesting that orchidectomy, or oestrogen administration, may cause regression of metastases.

Corticosteroids also have a place in the management of breast cancer. Not only do they cause regression of tumour in a small percentage of cases, but they are useful in the management of complications such as hypercalcaemia. They may also be used as part of a combination chemotherapy regime.

Prostate Cancer

The early animal work suggested that this tumour could be subject to hormonal manipulation. Clinical studies have confirmed that there is a proportion of patients who respond, but that survival rates are not increased significantly. Stilboestrol (1 mg t.i.d.) is the treatment usually recommended. However, it has become clear, even at this low dose, that significant side effects may occur. This is especially the case as the population at risk is an elderly group, with co-existing cardiovascular disease. There is an increased mortality from coronary heart disease and stroke. However, significant improvement occurs in a group of patients, and the quality of life is maintained.

Endometrial Cancer

Cancer of the body of uterus (adenocarcinoma) is not a particularly common neoplasm. Consequently large studies on the effectiveness of hormone therapy have not been performed. However, there is enough epidemiological data (increased incidence of endometrial cancer in patients taking oestrogens) and biochemical data (presence of progesterone receptors in tumours) to suggest that the neoplasm may respond to the progestogens. Clinical trials have indicated some benefit and several commercial preparations are available for oral or intramuscular use.

Renal Cancer

Sufficient clinical data is available to indicate that, in a small percentage of cases, metastatic renal cancer responds to the use of progestational agents. Medroxyprogesterone (Provera) has been the drug most frequently used, at a dose of 100 mg three times per day. No well-conducted controlled clinical trials have conclusively demonstrated its efficacy.

Lymphomas

Although this term covers a wide range of neoplastic conditions, it has been shown, with most histological variations, that corticosteroids are effective drugs in the treatment of these conditions. Prednisolone is part of the MOPP regime, and forms part of many chemotherapeutic schedules.

Leukaemias

Again corticosteroids have demonstrated their usefulness in the remission induction of acute lymphoblastic leukaemia, usually in association with a cytotoxic drug. In some chronic leukaemias corticosteroids also have a place in management.

Myeloma

Corticosteroids, in conjunction with melphelan, are the standard method of initial treatment of this tumour. It has been shown that the addition of prednisolone increases the responsiveness.

OTHER USES OF STEROID HORMONES

In addition to being used specifically as anti-tumour treatment these hormones may also be used in the supportive care of the patient.

Anorexia

This difficult symptom to control may respond to the use of prednisolone given in small doses which increases appetite and induces a feeling of well-being. The anabolic steroids have also been used for this purpose.

Hypercalcaemia

The presence of a raised serum calcium and the symptoms associated with this (p. 94) may respond dramatically to the use of prednisolone. Other methods may also be required to control this problem.

Brain Metastases

When brain metastases are present and associated with symptoms of raised intracranial pressure, corticosteroids, usually dexamethazone, may reduce this, and improve overall performance.

Adrenal Failure

Tumour involvement of the adrenal may result in adrenal failure. Although it is likely that no significant anti-tumour effect will occur, the use of corticosteroids may improve the patient symptomatically.

The use of corticosteroids in septic shock still remains controversial but most investigators believe that they do have a part to play in the management of this problem.

Leukopenia, Anaemia and Thrombocytopenia

Both corticosteroids and androgens have been used to treat these haematological complications of malignancy. Where leukopenia is associated with the use of chemotherapy the anabolic or androgenic steroids may protect the marrow against the effects of the drugs. It has been suggested that androgens stimulate stem cells and so improve the anaemia of malignancy. This, however, is a complex problem and one which requires further investigations.

SIDE EFFECTS OF STEROID HORMONES

The indiscriminate use of steroids may be associated with significant side effects.

(1) *Oestrogens*. Nausea and fluid retention. Gynaecomastia and hyperpigmentation. Cardiovascular problems including coronary thrombosis and stroke may occur. Hypercalcaemia may be induced when bone metastases are present.

(2) *Androgens*. Virilisation, with increased hair growth. Obstructive jaundice may occur with some drugs.

(3) *Progestational agents*. Fluid retention and occasional nausea.

(4) *Corticosteroids*. Fluid retention, hypertension, cushingoid facies, osteoporosis, mild diabetes, infection and gastrointestinal bleeding.

THE USE OF NON-STEROIDAL HORMONES IN THE MANAGEMENT OF CANCER

There is no doubt that the steroid hormones have an important part to play in the management of cancer. The non-steroidal hormones, however, have only a limited role at present. Some hormones have been used to monitor progress of the disease, such as the gonadotrophin levels in choriocarcinoma. Others have been used to study hormonal relationships in particular cancers. This is the case in breast cancer where the role of pituitary hormones such as prolactin are being defined at present. Insulin tolerance tests have been used to assess pituitary function after hypophysectomy.

The only non-steroidal hormones which have been used in a therapeutic way are adenocorticotrophic hormone (ACTH) and thyroxine. ACTH has been used in the same way as corticosteroids, with, if anything, fewer side effects. Thyroxine has been used in the treatment of thyroid neoplasms. It is considered likely that the control of neoplastic growth of the thyroid is related to the presence of thyroid stimulating hormone (TSH). Following thyroidectomy or radiation to the tumour, continuous thyroxine inhibits TSH release and good long-term remissions have been obtained. Thyroxine has also been used in the treatment of breast cancer though no controlled trials have shown its value. It is not indicated in the present management of breast cancer.

16 Immunotherapy

By a combination of clinical experience and laboratory data it has become evident that there is some form of host control over the development and spread of cancer. This information has come from several sources and is of three broad types.

CLINICAL EVIDENCE OF A HOST RESPONSE TO HUMAN TUMOURS

This includes the facts that cancers may occasionally undergo spontaneous regression, and that following resection of the primary tumour, metastatic disease may disappear. There are also the clinical observations of the waxing and waning of metastatic deposits suggesting that the host can in some way control growth rates of tumours. In addition there is the observation that some patients may survive for very long periods of time without evidence of neoplasms, and subsequently, very rapidly, develop widespread disease suggesting sudden loss of host control. Similarly, some responses to chemotherapy are much more pronounced than would be expected and might indicate that a host mechanism is involved. This is the case with choriocarcinoma and Burkitt's lymphoma. It has been noted that at post mortem the prevalence of some tumours, e.g. thyroid and prostatic cancer, is much higher than would be expected clinically. It has been implied as a result that the host is capable of eliminating a number of small tumours. Histological examination of draining lymph nodes has shown that the presence of a neoplasm may stimulate the changes associated with antigenic challenge and such a finding is associated with a good prognosis. Finally it has been observed that there is a higher incidence of cancer in patients with immunodeficiency, either primary or secondary. The primary immunodeficiency diseases are rare though secondary immunodeficiency due to the administration of drugs, e.g. following immunosuppression for renal transplantation, is more common (see p. 72–3).

EVIDENCE FROM EXPERIMENTAL ANIMALS

Once pure inbred strains of animals became available for experimental studies, it was possible to demonstrate not only that most tumours were antigenic and elicited both a humoral and cell mediated immune response, but that the development and growth of neoplasms could often be controlled by immunological methods. Thus the development of cancers could be prevented by the use of specific vaccines and the tumours themselves could be made to regress when given immunotherapy of various sorts. The identification of serum factors (blocking factors) which can interfere with the effectiveness of the cell-mediated immune response has been an important conceptual advance.

ANTIGENICITY OF HUMAN TUMOURS

Evidence has now accumulated to indicate that some human tumours are very weakly antigenic in that an immune response, whether humoral or cell mediated, can be detected against the specific tumour. These facts, in addition to the results obtained from a number of clinical trials of immunotherapeutic procedures, have suggested that the ability to modulate and manipulate the immune response in cancer patients may be clinically useful.

THE AIMS OF CLINICAL IMMUNOTHERAPY

The first and chief aim of clinical immunotherapy must be to so modify the existing immune response against the tumour that the effector arm of the immune response, either humoral or cell mediated, destroys cancer cells. This may be achieved in several ways. The host may be stimulated, by specific or non-specific methods, to produce an enhanced response. Alternatively the immune response may be temporarily improved by transferring serum or cells to the patient from another individual or animal which has been sensitised to the tumour. Finally a method to eliminate blocking factors may be employed (see p. 71).

The second aim of immunotherapy must be to use the information obtained during therapy to understand more about the immune response in cancer and to determine, in individual patients, which components are most important.

The third aim must be to establish the safety and effectiveness of the various methods employed. It is insufficient to know that in a highly artificial situation, as with an inbred mouse strain and an antigenic transplantable tumour, that immunotherapy can control the growth of the tumour. The requirements are carefully controlled clinical trials in which the dosage, route, safety and effectiveness of the procedure are all recorded. Immunotherapy is in its infancy and clinical evidence of its effectiveness either alone or in combination with other modalities of therapy is still required.

METHODS OF IMMUNOTHERAPY

Immunotherapy may either be specific or non-specific, active or passive (table 16.1). Specific immunotherapy means that the therapy is directed against the individual tumour. Non-specific immunotherapy implies that the immune

Table 16.1 Immunotherapy methods

	Active	*Passive*
Specific	Tumour cell extracts	Sensitised cells
	Tumour vaccines	Serum
Non-specific	BCG	White cell transfusions
	C. parvum	Serum factors
	Levamisole	

response is stimulated in a general way, no attempt being made to tailor this to a particular tumour. Active immunotherapy is concerned with the direct stimulation of the immune response, while with passive immunotherapy cells or sera are transferred from another source to the patient with the tumour. There are many combinations of immunotherapy and these are now described.

Non-specific Active Immunotherapy

Many methods have been used to stimulate the immune response in a non-specific way. At the present time, however, only three methods are regularly in use.

(1) Bacille Calmette Guerin (BCG) is the most widely used method. The BCG may be given into the tumour (intralesional) or into the skin by scarification at a site distant to the neoplasm. A range of immunological responses is stimulated by BCG. Several strains of BCG have been used. In each case live, attenuated organisms are employed.

(2) *Corynebacterium parvum* (*C. parvum*) is given as a killed suspension of organisms and is administered either subcutaneously or intravenously. The reticulo-endothelial system is stimulated following administration.

(3) Levamisole is a compound, originally designed as an antihelminthic agent, which was found, incidentally, to have the property of stimulating the immune response. Numerous clinical trials of its effectiveness are now under-way. Levamisole is given orally.

Although these compounds are the most frequently used numerous other chemical and biological agents have been employed. These included a range of bacterial toxins and extracts, viruses live and killed, and chemicals such as dinitrochlorobenzene (DNCB).

Non-specific Passive Immunotherapy

This is the least frequently used method at the present time. It includes the use of allogenic white cells or white cell fractions and serum fractions from normal individuals or from individuals bearing similar forms of tumour. No consistently reproducible results have been obtained by these methods.

Specific Active Immunotherapy

This technique is perhaps the most attractive conceptually. It implies that the patients own immune response is stimulated specifically. To do this, tumour extracts, irradiated whole tumour cells or cells killed by other methods have been used. In some instances live tumour cells have been used though the ethics of this must be questioned. The tumour cell vaccine may be given alone, or with the addition of non-specific methods such as BCG or *C. parvum*. Although promising, few studies have demonstrated any substantial benefit.

Specific Passive or Adoptive Immunotherapy

With this technique a secondary host is specifically stimulated by a tumour vaccine of one sort or another. Sensitised lymphoid cells or serum are then transferred to the patient donating the tumour. In most instances the secondary host is an animal, goat, pig or monkey, though humans have been employed. At the present time this technique has little to offer.

CLINICAL APPLICATION OF IMMUNOTHERAPY

In spite of a great deal of work over the past 50 years it is still difficult to place immunotherapy in proper perspective in relation to other forms of cancer therapy. There have been so many promising lines of attack which seem to have floundered when put to the test. A large number of individual case reports have been published indicating a therapeutic advantage by using immunotherapy. Few larger trials have convincingly demonstrated its value, though results remain encouraging enough to continue investigation.

One of the problems with immunotherapy is that it has been used in patients with very advanced disease, in spite of the fact that most of the animal work has demonstrated that it is most effective in cases where the number of tumour cells is small. More information is required on patients with minimal tumour mass. Most of the exciting results have been reported where chemotherapy or surgery have reduced tumour bulk, to be followed by immunotherapy. This has been demonstrated, though not conclusively, in the acute leukaemias and in malignant melanoma.

This section has dealt with the use of immunotherapy as a single modality. However, it may play an important role when used in combination with chemotherapy. Several studies have now indicated that the combination of both modalities is superior to either alone. This has been reported in colonic cancer, breast cancer, acute leukaemia, malignant melanoma, lung cancer and ovarian cancer. In most cases non-specific immunotherapy has been used.

A much more interesting combination is the use of tumour specific antibodies coupled to chemotherapeutic drugs. It is suggested that the antibodies 'home' to the tumour and the drug is then released. This would be truly specific chemotherapy and is akin to the notion of the 'magic bullet'. Early work in this field has at least given hope for the future. This will be discussed in a later section.

COMPLICATIONS OF IMMUNOTHERAPY

It is frequently implied that even if immunotherapy does no good it certainly does no harm. This is not the case and there is no better way of destroying the reputation of immunotherapy than by its indiscriminate application. The complications associated with immunotherapy may be divided into general problems and those associated with an altered immunological state.

BCG, for example, if given intralesionally or intradermally may result in the development of an indolent discharging ulcer which may be painful and cause considerable stress to the patient. BCG is composed of viable though attenuated organisms, and in patients with already compromised immunological function systemic infections with mycobacteria may occur. In addition a granulomatous hepatitis has been reported, and transient abnormalities in liver function recorded.

C. parvum may also be associated with the development of local painful lesions when given subcutaneously. However, its main side effect is the development of severe systemic reactions, worse when given intravenously than subcutaneously. The patient may develop an elevated temperature and be subjected to severe rigors.

From an immunological angle the stimulation of the immune response may have several adverse effects. Immune complexes may be formed and systemic effects on joint and renal function noted. More importantly, however, 'blocking' factors in the serum may be produced and enhanced tumour growth occur.

This list of complications is given to stimulate a note of caution in the often haphazard use of immunotherapy.

17 Other Methods of Treating Cancer

Over the next few years it is likely that with increasing knowledge and skill, the results of treatment with the established forms of cancer therapy (surgery, radiotherapy, chemotherapy, hormone therapy and immunotherapy) will improve. There are, however, several other forms of treatment which are still being evaluated or have already a role in cancer therapy, which do not fit into the above categories. The place of these methods of treatment still remains to be defined.

CRYOSURGERY

It has been known for sometime that if tissues are frozen to a sufficiently low temperature the cells involved will die. It was logical, therefore, to try this form of treatment in the cancer patient. The tissue is frozen by applying a probe, the tip of which is cooled to a very low temperature by liquid nitrogen or by the Joule–Thomson effect. The tissue is frozen until an 'ice-ball' is formed and then allowed to warm to body temperature. The use of cryosurgery in benign lesions of the cervix, bladder and anal region has been well described. In patients with cancer it has been used in tumours of the head and neck, in the treatment of locally recurrent breast disease, and in prostatic cancer. It is an acceptable method of therapy in these tumours, and is subject to the same limitations as surgery.

INTERFERON

This compound is produced when a virus infects an individual patient, or indeed cells in culture. The material has been isolated and found to be chemically a protein with a molecular weight of 15 000–20 000. It has the property of being able to protect cells and human volunteers against infection by certain viruses but it is time consuming and expensive to produce and has only been evaluated in the treatment of a limited number of neoplasms. It appears to be effective, in the short term, in the prevention of metastasis formation in osteosarcoma. However, many more trials are required. Interferon may well be of use in the future, and it would appear to have the added advantage of safety of administration.

TRANSFER FACTOR

Some years ago Sherwood Lawrence described a soluble factor, which could be isolated from sensitised leucocytes, and which, when transferred into non-sensitised individuals, could confer immunity. The initial clinical work was performed on patients with infectious disease and immunity was transferred from one patient to another. Its role in the treatment of chronic muco-cutaneous candidiasis has been fully studied. It has also been given to a wide variety of cancer patients with some evidence of action. However, it is impossible to say, at the present time, whether transfer factor will have any part to play in the management of the cancer patient.

HYPERTHERMIA

It has been established, in animal studies, that increasing the body temperature to a few degrees above normal may selectively kill cancer cells. In addition, the use of other treatments such as radiotherapy or chemotherapy while the animal is at a higher than normal body temperature, may enhance the effect of these therapies. In patients with cancer similar results have been reported. Patients are anaesthetised and the body temperature elevated to 40–41°C. This has been evaluated in conjunction with other treatment modalities and results have been encouraging. Special expertise is required to perform the technique and more work is required before the role of hyperthermia in the treatment of cancer can be defined.

LIPOSOMES AND DRUG CARRIERS

While this technique may be considered to be an extension of the use of chemotherapy it is possible that non-chemotherapeutic agents, e.g. radioactive compounds or bacterial toxins, may also be used, and so it is considered separately. The use of such vehicles is based on the fact that neoplastic cells may have altered membrane properties and so appear capable of taking up particles more rapidly than normal cells.

It is possible to construct very small liquid spheres, liposomes, and to place inside these spheres chemotherapeutic drugs, radioactive isotopes or other toxic compounds. The hypothesis is that these loaded liposomes will be taken up by the cancer cell and, because of the enclosed drug or toxin, the cell will be killed. The available experimental evidence suggests that the idea may be feasible and may increase the selectivity of anticancer agents. In addition to the use of liposomes, deoxyribonucleic acid has been used as a carrier in conjunction with adriamycin. The use of drugs in combination with tumour specific antibody is described elsewhere.

MISCELLANEOUS METHODS

For many years now literally hundreds of new methods of treating cancer have been described. These include the use of toxins, sera, vitamin preparations, plant products and many other substances. While none has been shown in a clinical trial setting to be more effective than conventional therapy, the occasional responses obtained give food for thought.

18 The Multimodality Approach to Cancer Therapy

The individual methods of treatment have now been described. However, it is unusual nowadays for a single method to be employed in the treatment of any particular tumour. Rather, there is increasing use of two or more modalities of cancer therapy in any one patient. For some tumours there is a well-defined sequence of treatments, e.g. surgery – radiotherapy – chemotherapy. For other cancers, treatments are given in a less organised way, a change of treatment being made when a clinically significant event occurs, e.g. the development of metastatic disease. One aim of cancer therapy should be to define the use and timing of each modality in the treatment of individual cancers, and to combine these in a rational way. Thus the concept of treatment planning may be introduced; a concept that implies a knowledge of the natural history of cancer, the mode of spread in individual tumours, and the values and limitations of each form of therapy.

The use of combined modality therapy assumes that a group of clinicians and paramedical workers, the cancer care team, decide on treatment policies for individual tumours and develop an integrated cancer treatment service. The necessity to evaluate treatment becomes even more crucial when several methods of therapy are being used. The accurate recording of data and the reporting of results forms a necessary part of the combined modality approach.

There are two basic aspects to this approach which require discussion. These are the selection of the initial modality of therapy, and the concept of minimal tumour mass.

INITIAL MODALITY OF TREATMENT

It is standard practice, at least in the solid tumours, that the bulk of the tumours, or as much as possible, be removed surgically. While this may be the correct initial therapy for carcinoma of stomach, pancreas, colon or lung, its use may be challenged. This is particularly the case in those tumours with poor survival rates, in which a new approach to therapy is required. This does not diminish the value of surgery, it simply alters its timing. Again, with several tumours radiotherapy is given immediately post-operatively. In most instances this reduces the incidence of local recurrence, but may not contribute to an increase in survival. It may be more important to use radiotherapy pre-operatively, or late in the disease to deal with bulk tumours. Chemotherapy in solid tumours has been traditionally reserved for advanced, metastatic disease. Yet a consideration of the effectiveness of chemotherapy would indicate that it is much more useful when the tumour mass is small.

The same conditions apply to the use of immunotherapy. There is thus a tendency to use chemotherapy earlier in the natural history of the disease. These remarks are not intended to upset the traditional methods of treating solid tumours. Rather, that they should stimulate a closer look at the management of each individual neoplasm. It is not unreasonable to postulate that carcinoma of the lung be treated by chemotherapy first, followed by surgery to remove bulk tumour, then by radiotherapy to deal with those areas where tumour has been left behind. The survival rate for lung cancer is at present so poor that a change in management may be necessary to improve results. It is recognised, however, that the design and execution of clinical trials will be required to explore these possibilities and it may be several years before the optimum combination of treatment can be made. Several of the results, described later, will show how long it may take to answer such questions.

A further point which may be made in relation to the timing of therapy is the exact nature of the treatment to be used in combination with other modalities. Thus, in cancer of the breast, it may be said that the choice of operation does not influence survival if surgery is used as the sole modality of therapy. However, this may *not* be the case when surgery is combined with other forms of therapy. The choice of operation may be extremely important.

THE TREATMENT OF MINIMAL TUMOUR MASS

With increasing understanding of tumour growth kinetics, and the increasing effectiveness of chemotherapy, it has become important to consider the management of the patient who has had the bulk of his tumour treated either by surgery or radiotherapy. Following removal of the main mass of the tumour the clinician has two choices: (1) to leave the patient without further therapy and await recurrence or the development of metastases; (2) to add another modality of treatment at the time when tumour mass is small.

The choice depends on the individual tumour, its mode of spread and the overall survival rate. Thus with carcinoma of the breast, with no histologically involved nodes and no evidence of distant spread the survival rate is high, over 80 per cent at five years. It might be considered by the clinician that the addition of further therapy to such patients would be unhelpful. On the other hand if lymph nodes are involved, even though they have been removed, the prognosis is poor, less than 50 per cent five-year survival rate. In this case it might be considered important to add a second form of therapy.

It is clearly important that the side effects of such treatments are minimised if chemotherapy is given as an adjunct to surgery when the tumour bulk is small. It is also important, and indeed self-evident, that the chemotherapy used should be effective. It is usual to use those drugs which are effective in the treatment of advanced disease of the particular tumour.

The concept of treatment of minimal tumour mass has altered the approach to management of the cancer patient in several ways.

(1) It has become more important that the bulk of the tumour is removed, even if obvious macroscopic lesions are left behind. The chances of chemotherapy, immunotherapy or radiotherapy being helpful are increased if the tumour mass is small. The surgical operation performed may thus be of considerable importance.

(2) Chemotherapy, and to a lesser extent immunotherapy, is being used earlier in the disease. This has changed the outlook for several tumour types. Its more general application is theoretically attractive though caution should be exercised in the extrapolation of information, and in the widespread use of chemotherapy in early disease in all neoplasms.

(3) Because of the improved results obtained in a small number of responsive tumours, cancer, in general, is being treated more aggressively, and there is a greater sense of purpose and excitement in those treating cancer than in previous decades.

To illustrate the use of combined modality therapy, and the treatment of minimal tumour mass, several examples will be given. These have been chosen to highlight the important changes which have occurred recently. Many other trials of combined modality therapy in a whole range of tumours have been performed. Many have shown no advantage, or have been associated with a poorer survival. This does not negate the basic concept, it simply shows how difficult it may be to choose the correct treatment, and to combine it appropriately with other therapies. The results that follow will be described in relation to individual tumours, and are not tied to modalities of therapy. They are to be regarded only as examples of the concept and not as definite essays on the therapy of particular tumours.

Wilm's Tumour

The treatment of this tumour is an excellent example of combined modality therapy. Using surgery alone a 30 per cent two-year survival rate can be obtained. By the addition of post-operative radiotherapy the rate is increased to 44 per cent. If the disease is then left until metastases occur, the addition of chemotherapy results in no real benefit. However, if the chemotherapy is given at the time when tumour mass is small, i.e. following radiotherapy, then the two-year survival rate is increased to over 80 per cent. This striking example of combined modality therapy also highlights one of its major problems: the time factor. The results obtained above, have been the result of over thirty years experience of treating this disease.

Rectal Carcinoma

When treated by abdominoperineal resection, this tumour has around a 30 per cent five-year survival rate. When, in addition to surgery, the patient is given pre-operative radiotherapy at dosages of 500–2000 rads, there is an increase in the five-year survival rate to over 45 per cent. The pre-operative radiotherapy has no adverse effect on wound healing or on post-operative complications. Pre-operative radiotherapy has been used in a number of other tumours, though in most instances its role remains to be defined.

Acute Leukaemia

In childhood leukaemia the survival rate at five years has increased from nil to over 60 per cent in the last ten years. This has occurred because of the introduction of effective drugs, the use of combination chemotherapy and, most importantly, well-designed clinical trials. However, as increasingly long survival rates become the norm other complications have developed, notably the high incidence of meningeal leukaemia. The drugs used in induction therapy do not cross the blood brain barrier regularly, and do not prevent dissemination of the disease in the meninges. Accordingly it is necessary to use other forms of therapy, in this case radiotherapy, to improve the overall survival rate. Radiotherapy to the brain in combination with intrathecal cytotoxic drugs is given, so preventing the development of meningeal disease. This is an example of combined modality therapy in a disease which is treated predominantly with chemotherapy.

In chronic myeloid leukaemia there is some evidence that splenectomy may improve prognosis and facilitate treatment with chemotherapy. Although this may be disputed it shows how a third form of treatment may be integrated into planned therapy. It also indicates the value of full assessment of any new procedure.

Breast Cancer

For many years now the standard treatment for cancer of the breast has been a mastectomy of one type or another, coupled with post-operative radiotherapy where indicated. The use of radiotherapy has reduced the incidence of local recurrence but there has been little effect on survival rates. More recently chemotherapy either with single agents or combinations of drugs has been used in the treatment of breast cancer with axillary node involvement. Initial results show that there is a reduction in the local and distant recurrence rates. It is too early to say whether or not there will be a significant effect on survival but the results are awaited with interest. Endocrine therapy in early breast cancer has been shown to prolong the disease free interval. For the present the role of endocrine therapy would appear to be predominantly in advanced disease.

Osteosarcoma and Ewings Tumour

These bony neoplasms are associated with very poor survival rates, usually less than 20 per cent at five years. The standard method of treatment involves surgical removal of the tumour followed by radiotherapy. Although local tumour control was often effective, these patients developed a very high incidence of pulmonary metastases. To overcome this problem, prophylactic radiotherapy to the lung fields has been used, but has not gained a great deal of ground. On the other hand, chemotherapy has been shown to delay the presentation of lung metastases and to improve survival rates. This shows clearly how the treatment of minimal tumour mass with effective therapy can indeed alter the prognosis and natural history of the disease.

Brain Tumours

These tumours are amongst the most difficult to control, and are associated with very low survival rate. In recent years the combination of surgery, whole brain irradiation and chemotherapy has improved the survival rate to a small degree. Although this has not been dramatic it illustrates the point that it may take several years before the correct sequence of modalities is developed.

Malignant Melanoma

This is a notoriously difficult tumour to treat because of the wide variation in its natural history. However, it has recently been shown that a combination of chemotherapy and immunotherapy in patients who have lymph node involvement improves survival rate. Adequate excision of the primary tumour is of great importance.

Testicular Tumours

Seminomas are treated with the combined modalities of surgery and radiotherapy. They are particularly responsive to radiation and excellent long-term responses can be obtained. Teratomas, on the other hand, are less responsive but the increasing use of the three major modalities, in combination, has given encouraging results. Chemotherapy may be used prior to radiotherapy, the radiation being used to deal with residual tumour.

The Lymphomas

This broad group of neoplastic diseases has benefited considerably by the use of more than one modality of therapy. In particular, radiotherapy and chemotherapy have been used together. As experience increases, so the relative role and timing of these two methods of therapy are changing. These modifications occur in response to carefully conducted trials on the merits of treatment in different stages and histological appearances of the tumour.

Future Developments

It is likely that there will be an overall improvement in cancer treatment by the integration of different modalities of therapy. The standard combinations of surgery, chemotherapy and radiotherapy are being actively explored at the present time in most tumour types. The combinations of immunotherapy and chemotherapy, and hormone therapy and chemotherapy, represent growing points in this area.

IMMUNOCHEMOTHERAPY

This may be developed in two ways. First, the combination of chemotherapy with the non-specific immunostimulants such as BCG, *Corynebacterium parvum* or Levamisole. Several clinical trials at present indicate that this type of combined modality therapy may be of considerable value in lung cancer, colonic cancer, malignant melanoma and ovarian cancer. More information is required on each of these tumours. The second way in which immunotherapy could be used would be to combine cytotoxic drugs with tumour specific antibody, the drug–antibody complex allowing greater selectivity. Animal experimental work has indicated that this possibility may be realised, though it is clear that direct drug–antibody conjugation may not be required. Clinical trials with the use of drug–antibody complexes are inconclusive at present.

HORMONE AND DRUG THERAPY

Hormones, in general, act by reducing the growth fraction of the tumour. Thus a combination of drugs and hormones might at first sight appear contradictory in that chemotherapeutic agents are more effective when there is a high growth fraction. It may be that this can be used to advantage, as release from hormone therapy may increase the number of cells in division and chemotherapy, given at that point, may be more effective. A great deal more must be learned about tumour kinetics, and the value of cell synchronisation, before this aspect of combined modality therapy becomes feasible.

19 Cancer in Children

Cancer is the second leading cause of death in childhood, accidents being the most common cause. The pattern of neoplasms which develop is different from the adult situation, there being a preponderance of embryonal tumours and leukaemias (table 19.1). The common epithelial adult neoplasms, such as lung, breast or gastrointestinal cancer are not usually seen in childhood.

Table 19.1 Common sites of cancer in children under 15 years. (American Cancer Society)

	%
Leukaemia	37
Brain and CNS	21
Lymphomas	10
Kidney	8
Bone	5
Connective tissue	3
Other	16
	100

AETIOLOGY

There is a peak of incidence of cancer in early childhood, suggesting that some of the factors which initiate the development of the disease occur *in utero*, or are genetically associated.

Transplacental carcinogenesis is a well-recognised event in animal models. It has been established in humans that the use of stilboestrol during pregnancy is associated with an increased risk of development of vaginal cancer in female children. Exposure of the foetus to x-rays during pregnancy is also associated with an increased risk of developing childhood cancer.

There also appears to be an association between certain congenital syndromes and leukaemia. This is the case with Down's syndrome, Bloom's syndrome or Fanconi's aplastic anaemia. Each of these conditions is associated with chromosomal instability or fragility (chapter 6). Children who have immunodeficiency disease also have an increased risk of developing cancer. It has also been postulated that other factors, as yet unknown, act *in utero* causing genetic changes which subsequently result in the development of cancer.

Viruses have been associated with the development of leukaemias in animals and birds (chapter 5). As yet, there is no direct evidence that they cause leukaemia in children but there is interesting epidemiological data suggesting that clusters of cases of leukaemia may be found together. This time-space association may suggest an 'infectious cause' but the data have not been fully confirmed, and no causative virus has been isolated from leukaemia cells.

The pathology of childhood tumours is often difficult, and requires special expertise. For this reason the advice of the pathologist should be sought wherever possible.

THE CLINICAL PRESENTATION OF CANCER IN CHILDHOOD

The child may be born with an obvious mass or neoplasm. In this case treatment may be started immediately. However, the child may present with vague symptoms, or no symptoms at all. Every opportunity should be taken to examine children and abnormalities investigated. The presentation may be misleading in that the child simply complains of malaise, weakness, fever, pallor or anorexia. Minor or major abnormalities may be noted in the peripheral blood. In all cases a 'high' incidence of suspicion should be retained.

THE MANAGEMENT OF CANCER IN CHILDHOOD

The management of the child with cancer follows exactly the same lines as in adults. Indeed many of the most exciting developments in cancer therapy have occurred in the childhood cancers, and the approach developed has been applied to adult cases.

There are, of course, technical difficulties to be overcome. The small size of infants makes repeated intravenous injections less feasible than in the adult. The control of bowel and bladder function in young children is not fully developed. This predisposes to an increased infection risk. There are also psychological problems in children who require barrier nursing or who require to make repeated visits to hospital.

The management of children with cancer is based on the principles of combined modality therapy and the integration of the cancer care team. Paediatric oncology groups have sprung up in most children's hospitals, and the advantages of children being treated by an experienced group must always be borne in mind. Several of the tumours in which effective treatment has been developed in recent years, the acute leukaemias, osteosarcoma, rhabdomyosarcoma etc, have been childhood neoplasms, and the task of management has been the integration of several methods of treatment.

The Role of the Cancer Care Team

Both the child and his family need careful consideration. The intensive treatment given to children with cancer nowadays may be associated with severe side effects. The parents should be kept fully informed of these, and of the prognosis of the child. The parents may require just as much support as the child. As childhood cancers are rare, a general practitioner may only see one or two in a lifetime. He too must be kept informed as to the changing management of the case and be encouraged to use the resources of the community to the full.

Table 20.1 Survival rates for various types of cancer

| Neoplasm | Sex | Survival rate (%) | | | | | |
| | | All stages | | Early | | Late | |
		5 years	10 years	5 years	10 years	5 years	10 years
Lip	M + F	69	48	72	51	38	24
Tongue	M + F	26	14	42	24	15	7
Salivary glands	M + F	79	69	88	78	34	25
Floor of mouth	M + F	35	19	52	31	23	11
Pharynx	M + F	20	12	33	20	18	9
Oesophagus	M + F	7	5	10	6	4	3
Stomach	M + F	9	6	30	19	10	6
Colon	M + F	36	24	58	40	33	22
Rectum	M + F	31	20	50	34	24	14
Liver	M + F	3	2	7	6	2	1
Gall bladder	M + F	8	6	27	19	5	4
Pancreas	M + F	3	1	5	5	2	1
Nasal cavities	M + F	33	20	40	29	26	17
Larynx	M + F	46	31	60	41	26	16
Lung	M + F	7	4	24	14	7	4
Epidermoid	(Surgically treatable) males	35					
Adenocarcinoma		20					
Large Cell		15					
Oat Cell		5					
Breast	F	54	37	73	55	47	29
Cervix uteri	F	55	46	74	64	41	32
Body of uterus	F	63	52	75	62	44	34
Ovary	F	29	22	67	55	33	23
Vulva	F	50	35	61	44	35	23
Vagina	F	29	23	40	37	28	16
Prostatic	M	34	15	42	19	35	15
Testis	M	62	57	80	74	59	55
Seminoma	M	85	80	–	–	–	–
Teratoma	M	55	40	–	–	–	–
Kidney	M + F	30	20	52	36	26	16
Bladder	M + F	42	27	52	34	16	10
Melanoma of skin	M + F	54	45	70	58	35	27
Eye	M + F	71	59	76	63	47	41
Brain	M + F	26	20	28	22	18	14
Thyroid	M + F	76	70	89	83	77	70
Bone	M + F	32	25	45	38	28	19
Connective tissue sarcoma	M + F	44	35	62	51	31	22
Reticulum cell sarcoma	M + F	14	9	–	–	–	–

Table 20.1 (*continued*)

Neoplasm	Sex	Survival rate (%)					
		All stages		Early		Late	
		5 years	10 years	5 years	10 years	5 years	10 years
Non-Hodgkin's lymphoma	M + F	25	13	–	–	–	–
Hodgkin's disease Diagnosed 1940–49	M + F	25	14	–	–	–	–
Diagnosed 1950–59	M + F	34	22	–	–	–	–
Diagnosed 1960–64	M + F	42	36	–	–	–	–
Diagnosed 1965–69	M + F	60	–	–	–	–	–
Diagnosed 1970–74	M + F	75	–	–	–	–	–
Multiple myeloma	M + F	7	3	–	–	–	–
Acute lymphocytic leukaemia 1940–49	M + F	–	–	–	–	–	–
1950–59	M + F	1	–	–	–	–	–
1960–64	M + F	3	–	–	–	–	–
1965–69	M + F	15	–	–	–	–	–
1970–74	M + F	60	–	–	–	–	–
Acute myeloid leukaemia	M + F	1	–	–	–	–	–
Chronic lymphocutic leukaemia	M + F	29	–	–	–	–	–
Chronic myeloid leukaemia	M + F	11	2	–	–	–	–

terms this definition is of little value. It is sometimes stated that a patient who has survived at least fifteen years after diagnosis, and who remains tumour free, may be considered to be cured. However, it is known that although survival curves may approach, or be equal to those of a normal population, there is still a chance of developing recurrent disease. Cure is a word which should be used very cautiously in relation to cancer.

A great deal of the information required for these studies comes from the Cancer Registries. These registries function to collect data for further investigation of national and international patterns of disease. It is imperative that the doctor appreciates the value of such registries and co-operates in every way to maintain a high standard of reporting.

Part 4

The Cancer Patient and the Community

20 The Results of Cancer Treatment

It is often stated that there have been no improvements in the overall survival rate for cancer in the past 30 years. While this may have some vestige of truth it does hide many of the changes which have occurred in individual cancers. It also takes no account of the changing patterns of disease incidence, or the newer methods of treatment which have been recently introduced.

SURVIVAL RATES FOR VARIOUS NEOPLASMS

In documenting treatment results, and survival rates, it is common to use five-year and ten-year survival figures (table 20.1). Such figures, however, have limitations, for example, the five-year survival rates indicate only that the patient is alive, but not that he is free of disease. The purpose of this chapter is to draw together survival rates for various types of cancer in order that some index of prognosis can be given for each type of cancer. The figures come from a variety of sources and are intended to give an overall impression of the survival rate of the particular neoplasm. Where possible results have been divided into those obtained when early cancers or late cancers are treated. As the histological type of cancer may be important this is also included for some neoplasms. It should be noted that to obtain ten-year survival figures, treatment must have been carried out prior to this. Thus changes in treatment in the last ten years would not influence these figures. Where there is no significant change in survival rates between males and females, both are combined.

From the results noted in table 20.1, crude as they may be, several conclusions can be drawn.

(1) The earlier the diagnosis is made, the better the overall survival rate.

(2) There are important variations in survival rate with histology, e.g. testicular tumours, lung tumours, and the lymphomas.

(3) Where accurate data are available, it appears that there has been a progressive increase in the survival rate with several tumours. Examples of such tumours recorded here are Hodgkin's disease and the leukaemias.

It has been stated that in the 1930s one patient in five survived at least five years following the diagnosis of cancer. By the 1960s this became one in three and in the 1970s at least one patient in every two with the diagnosis of cancer will survive for at least five years. This may not seem a great achievement, but it is a step in the right direction.

The concept of 'cure' is one which is frequently raised in relation to cancer statistics; 'cure' may be defined in several ways, none of which is particularly satisfactory. A cure can only really be established by the failure to detect tumour in a patient at autopsy some years after the diagnosis. In clinical

21 The Cancer Care Team

The patient with cancer is not an isolated individual, living within a hospital ward or making regular visits to an out-patient clinic. He is part of the community where he lives with his family. He is employed in the community, and makes use of community resources. To consider the cancer patient as part of the community opens up new vistas for the management of such patients and adds further dimensions to the cancer problem. To visualise the cancer patient as part of the community means looking less at the individual problem and more at the overall impact of cancer at a population level.

Consideration must be given to the total care required by such patients, and the role of the cancer care team in the community. This team must be concerned with epidemiological problems, screening and early diagnosis, public education and the logistics of cancer care. Such factors, often considered to be less exciting than the most recent developments in molecular biology or the newest form of immunotherapy, nevertheless may contribute greatly to the overall problem of cancer and assist in improving the care of a large number of patients.

COMPOSITION OF THE TEAM

Over the past few years the concept of the cancer care team has developed to include not only the wide variety of medical specialists involved but nursing staff, paramedical workers, basic scientists and the clergy. This team, working in an integrated way meets the very complex needs of the cancer patient. The team approach became necessary as the requirement to consider the *whole* patient became more apparent. It seems obvious that the cancer patient should be considered, not as 'the case of gastric cancer in bed 17', but as an individual, with individual requirements and problems. These secondary problems of a social or psychological nature are often just as troublesome to the patient and may require just as much attention as the tumour itself. The team, however, must have a leader. This is necessary, not only in order that decisions should be made, but that the patient knows whom to contact and discuss problems. Thus although a whole variety of people may be involved in care it is essential that the progress of the patient is reviewed regularly by a relatively small group, easily identified by the patient. To make the best use of expertise, case review sessions in which individual patients are considered, problems identified and specialist help sought, are perhaps the most efficient methods of getting everyone together, making a decision and thereafter communicating that decision to the patient.

A very wide range of specialities are involved and each will be considered separately and their roles defined.

The Team Leader

This is usually a hospital-based doctor and he or she is primarily responsible for decisions to be made, specialist advice to be sought, treatment to be carried out and communication with the patient. The team leader in any particular patient may be any one of a wide variety of consultants from the medical oncologist, or the radiotherapist, to the general physician or surgeon. It does not matter a great deal which one actually heads the team as long as there is adherence to the concept of the team approach.

The General Practitioner

In the cancer care team the primary care physician holds a key position. He is the doctor of primary referral, responsible for sifting out those patients who require urgent investigation and treatment from those whose symptoms are related to non-malignant disease. He has a responsibility for health education, early diagnosis and screening in conjunction with other colleagues. Following hospital treatment the general practitioner is the lynch-pin around which subsequent care will rotate. He is responsible for the organisation of the community care of the patient including the tapping of community resources and the social services. He may be very concerned with the terminal care of the patient and the maintainance of continuity of care throughout the illness greatly facilitates management and makes the patient feel that someone does indeed care.

It is worth pointing out at this stage the enormous difference in the number of patients seen by the general practitioner and the hospital consultant. It has been estimated that each year a general practitioner will see five to six new cases of cancer. During this time the hospital consultant is likely to see between 100 and 125 new cancer patients.

The Nurse

The nurse remains a central figure in the care of the patient with cancer and in the past few years the role of the nurse has expanded considerably. No longer is she concerned only with the application of traditional nursing skills, but she has become involved with research projects and the treatment of patients. The various roles of the nurse in the cancer care team may be summarised as follows.

(1) As an observer. The nurse usually sees the patient more frequently than the doctor and can often comment more readily on pain control or symptom relief. She is able to observe more closely the ability of the patient to cope with eating, walking or just talking to other patients.

(2) As a research worker. The role of the nurse in this area is expanding rapidly. As an investigator of a clinical level, the nurse is now involved in

research projects such as those on drug metabolism, nutritional problems and social problems.

(3) As a communicator. Patients, and relatives, often find it easier to talk to a nurse and to tell her about their problems than to discuss them with a doctor. This is often the case with female patients who are able to relate more closely to the nurse. Conversely it is essential that the nurse is encouraged to discuss problems with patients and to use her own initiative in sitting down with patients and talking to them.

(4) Community nursing. This very rewarding branch of nursing is being increasingly utilised in the overall care of the cancer patient. The nurse becomes involved in the family situation and can co-ordinate symptom control with the general practitioner and the hospital. Night visiting services and domicillary nursing have allowed many more patients to be successfully treated at home.

(5) The nurse as a teacher. The experienced nurse has a tremendous amount to contribute by teaching other nurses and medical staff the skills she has learned.

The Health Visitor

The health visitor, based in the community or the hospital, is now seen as an important link in the chain of care of the patient with cancer. Not only is she concerned with continuing care but she has a basic role in health education.

Social Workers

Few cancer units could do without the expert support of an active social worker. When the whole patient is considered it is surprising how many of the problems which crop up have a social bearing, e.g. the lack of a telephone, the absence of an indoor toilet, no active caring relative, financial problems, provision of portable toilets or the provision of a meals-on-wheels service. The ramifications are considerable and the contribution made by the social worker is invaluable. It is often helpful to set aside time each week to discuss individual problems with the social worker in conjunction with other members of the cancer care team.

The Paramedical Staff

In a previous section the importance of rehabilitation of the cancer patient was emphasised. In this respect the physiotherapist, occupational therapist and speech therapist all have a role to play. With the active encouragement of these individuals the patient can often be made to feel better, become mobilised again and return home able to cope with the stresses and strains of family life. With the increasing use of drugs in the management of cancer it is essential that the pharmacist is brought into the team. In some areas the pharmacist may play a vital role in the care of the cancer patient.

The Scientist

The scientist, whether clinical or non-clinical, has a contribution to make to the care of the cancer patient. The basic scientist, immersed as he is in the intricacies of molecular biology, virology or immunology, must become aware of the clinical problems and in turn must be ready to communicate with his clinical colleagues on the nature of his own research work. This two-way process is essential if progress is to be made in the management of cancer.

Those scientists more associated with clinical work, pathologists, bacteriologists, physicists and epidemiologists, must also become involved in the cancer care team. Their involvement must not be superficial, rather they should be considered as an integral part of the team.

The Clergy

The religious beliefs of patients form an important part of the reaction of patients to illness and death. Many patients do have strong religious feelings and it is thus natural that they might require assistance of a minister or a priest. Such questions as the need to discuss theological problems with his or her religious advisor are difficult to raise, but must not be forgotten. Most hospitals have a chaplain and their contribution to the comfort of the patient is often underestimated.

TEAM MANAGEMENT

The team, as described, comprises a large number of individual members. In practice, however, where a single patient is concerned, the number is often small. What matters is that there is a wide range of expertise available which can be called upon when the situation demands it. Regular meetings of the whole team allow exchange of views and the development of management policies which can then be used to accumulate information on the most appropriate solutions to individual problems.

22 Epidemiology and the Prevention of Cancer

The prevention of cancer depends on the identification of carcinogenic agents, the detection of high risk groups and predisposing factors, and on a combination of screening techniques and public education. A multidisciplinary approach using the methodology of epidemiology, the advance in screening techniques and the utilisation of health education programmes is required. Various methods have been described for the prevention of cancer and they are reviewed in this chapter.

(1) *Social aspects.* Excessive cigarette smoking is associated with an increased risk of developing several forms of cancer. Excessive consumption of alcohol is associated with an increased risk of oral cancer, laryngeal, oesophageal, stomach and liver cancer.

(2) *Occupational factors.* These have been described in detail elsewhere (p. 35).

(3) *Dietary factors.* Epidemiological data suggests that dietary factors may be important in stomach and colonic cancer. As yet no definitive studies have shown that alteration of the diet will reduce the incidence of cancer but the use of a high roughage diet has been suggested as one way of reducing the incidence of colonic cancer.

(4) *Personal hygiene.* It is well known that circumcised males have a lower incidence of carcinoma of the penis than non-circumcised individuals. This has been related to inadequate removal of smegma in uncircumcised males. It has further been suggested that this may also be related to the higher incidence of carcinoma of the cervix in women whose partners have not been circumcised. Dental hygiene is also important in the prevention of oral cancers.

(5) *Viruses and cancers.* Although no conclusive evidence is yet available to implicate viruses in human cancer the possibility must always be borne in mind (p. 50).

(6) *Predisposing factors.* A wide range of high risk groups for individual cancers has been described. These are listed in table 22.1. It is suggested that individual patients who are under care for one of the factors listed have regular checks for the development of malignant disease. In some cases the risk becomes so high that prophylactic treatment may be considered. This is the case in ulcerative colitis where if the disease has been present for over 10 years then the risk of developing cancer is almost 20 times that of a normal population.

(7) *Drugs.* Several drugs have now been implicated in the increased incidence of various types of cancer. There may be adequate clinical indications

Table 22.1   Predisposing factors in human cancer

Site	Predisposing disease
Mouth } Vagina }	Leucoplakia
Oesophagus	Plummer—Vinson syndrome
Stomach	Achlorhydria, pernicious anaemia
Colon	Polyposis coli, ulcerative colitis, Gardner's syndrome
Small bowel	Peutz—Jegher's syndrome, Crohn's disease, coeliac disease
Liver	Cirrhosis
Testis	Cryptorchidism
Skin	Fair complexion, xeroderma pigmentosum
Leukaemia	Bloom's syndrome, Fanconi's anaemia
Bone sarcoma	Paget's disease
Various	Immunodeficiency disease, idiopathic or acquired

for giving patients such drugs, e.g. cytotoxic drugs in the treatment of cancer, but the risk must always be borne in mind (see table 4.1).

(8) *Skin markers of internal malignancy.* It is well documented that several skin lesions are associated with a higher incidence of internal malignances than would be expected. The mechanism for these changes is at present unknown. Skin diseases having an association with cancer include: Bowens disease, acanthosis nigricans, herpes zoster, acquired ichthyosis, Peutz—Jegher's syndrome, pruritus, erythroderma, dermatomyositis and thrombophlebitis. Paget's disease of nipple and vulva may also be considered.

With this very wide range of preventative measures available and with the increasing definition of high risk groups it becomes essential that this information is used to design effective screening techniques and to institute health education measures to increase public awareness of cancer prevention.

23 Early Diagnosis and Screening in Cancer Management

It is a prime aim of any cancer programme to prevent the occurrence of cancer. This, however, is not possible at the present time in the majority of tumours and it becomes essential to use a second line of attack, that of early detection. Unfortunately there is no simple, reliable method for detecting all forms of cancer, in spite of repeated claims to be able to do so.

One question to be raised is 'how early is early?' This will naturally depend on the type of tumour. A simple definition would be that early cancer is the smallest volume of tumour which can be detected by clinical or investigative methods. This, however, may be a large volume of tumour in terms of cell numbers. Thus one gram of tumour will contain 10^9 cells, or 1 billion cells and 1 milligram, 10^6 or 1 million cells. Thus even a 'small' tumour may be composed of 10^6–10^9 cells. It is not inconceivable, therefore, that some of these cells have become separated and have already spread throughout the body. Early detection may not therefore be equated with complete detection.

If cancer can be diagnosed early, and treated early, is this associated with an improved prognosis? It would seem reasonable to assume that this would be the case, and in almost all instances the earlier the treatment, the longer the survival. However, when the natural history of the tumour is considered it may be that this is not altered. In figure 23.1 tumour growth is shown

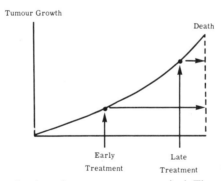

Figure 23.1   Effect of early or late treatment on survival. The survival is longer but there is no change in the natural history

diagrammatically, the growth increasing until death of the host occurs. It shows that early treatment is associated with a longer survival post-therapy than late treatment, though death occurs at the same time. However, if early treatment really alters the outlook (figure 23.2) then the patient survives longer than the predicted time of death and a true improvement has occurred. Sufficient data is now available in many tumours to indicate that early

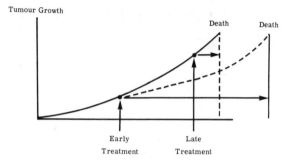

Figure 23.2   Effect of early or late treatment on survival. The survival is longer and there has been a definite change in the natural history

diagnosis and treatment alters the long-term outlook for the patient with cancer. In some forms of cancer, however, this has not been established with confidence.

The choice of the most appropriate population to be screened is of considerable importance. Should screening for various forms of cancer be available to the entire population or only to high or selected groups? In this connection the clues derived from epidemiological studies allow some selection of at risk population groups. Cancer of the cervix, for example, has a high risk group associated with women in the low income bracket, and with large families. This group, in particular, does not tend to support programmes designed to screen well-populations. A case can be made for screening the 'well-women' group or the equivalent 'mid-span' in men. Such programmes may be associated with screening for other forms of disease.

Screening procedures are costly in equipment and staff. For example, mammography or xeroradiotherapy require sophisticated equipment; cervical cytology necessitates trained medical and paramedical manpower to read the cytological preparations; and the cost of routine gastric endoscopy for stomach cancer is very great indeed. Although in theory, cost should not be a limiting factor, it does make it very necessary to justify the expense. A further limiting factor is the applicability of the screening procedure to large populations. Cervical cytology is a relatively simple procedure to organise on a large scale basis. Gastric endoscopy, on the other hand, is more difficult by an order of magnitude.

METHODS OF EARLY DIAGNOSIS AND SCREENING

Physical Examination

The clinical examination of the patient remains an integral part of any programme of early diagnosis. The examination is usually carried out by a doctor, but in special circumstances paramedical personnel, e.g. nurses, may be trained to perform a specific procedure. Examination of the breasts, general physical examination, and rectal examinations are carried out.

Self-examination

Breast lesions, in particular, may be detected by women trained to carry out this relatively simple procedure illustrated in figure 23.3 (a) to (e). The examination is performed monthly. Patients are also instructed to report any other abnormal finding such as alteration in bowel habit or abnormal bleeding.

Biochemical Examinations

There is no readily available test for detecting all types of cancer. Lactic dehydrogenase isozymes have been used and acid phosphatase levels are helpful in the diagnosis of prostatic cancer. Elevated serum immunoglobulin levels are useful in the diagnosis of myeloma. Simple techniques for the detection of occult blood in the stools or urine must never be forgotten.

Immunological Methods

It was hoped the oncofetal antigens (carcinoembryonic antigen (CEA, α-fetoprotein, etc)) which can be readily detected by radioimmunoassay would be useful in the early diagnosis of specific cancers. Measurement of CEA, for example, was initially considered to be specific for colonic cancer and hence would have met almost all the criteria for an effective screening method. However, subsequent investigation showed that true specificity was lacking. Other immunological tests, still in the process of being evaluated include the MEM test (macrophage electrophretic mobility), the SCM (structuredness of the cytoplasmic matrix) test. These tests depend on the presence of a population of sensitised lymphocytes in the peripheral blood of patients. They require further evaluation. The Makari test depends on a skin reaction to an intradermal tumour antigen challenge. Its importance is not yet known.

Radiological Techniques

The chest x-ray is naturally of great importance in cancer screening. The use of barium either as a meal or as an enema has been widely used in the detection of early gastrointestinal cancers. This is particularly the case when air-contrast x-rays are used. In the early detection of breast lesions mammography has been the most frequently used x-ray procedure. In this examination several views of the breast are taken. There has been some debate as to the safety of these procedures in relation to repeated screening, over exposure to radiation, and the induction of cancers of the breast. With

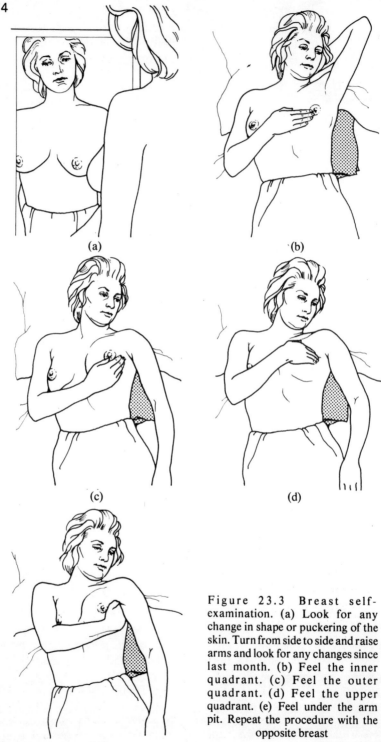

(a)

(b)

(c)

(d)

(e)

Figure 23.3 Breast self-examination. (a) Look for any change in shape or puckering of the skin. Turn from side to side and raise arms and look for any changes since last month. (b) Feel the inner quadrant. (c) Feel the outer quadrant. (d) Feel the upper quadrant. (e) Feel under the arm pit. Repeat the procedure with the opposite breast

high speed films now available the radiation risk is very small, but still measurable. Other radiological techniques such as xeroradiography and thermography have been evaluated in breast disease. Isotope scanning techniques have little place in the early detection of primary tumours at the present time though the development of such methods as gallium scanning may be of use in the long term. Scintiscan techniques however, have a place in the early diagnosis of secondary spread once the primary tumour has been identified.

Cytology

Even in the past few years there has been a considerable expansion in the role of cytology in screening and early diagnosis. Initially investigations were confined to the early detection of carcinoma of the uterine cervix. The 'pap test' (named after Dr G. Papanicolaou) is now widely used and large numbers of the population are regularly screened. The technique has many variations in obtaining the sample of the smear, and has been modified to use vaginal washings which can be obtained by the patient herself. Cytological methods are now used widely in the diagnosis of lung cancer. Aspiration cytology provides a relatively simple method of diagnosing breast lumps.

Endoscopy

The introduction of fiberoptic light systems has revolutionised the use of endoscopic methods. In the gastrointestinal tract, almost every region except small bowel can be visualised and, in conjunction with other methods such as biopsy and cytology, a high degree of accuracy in diagnosis can be achieved. Fiberoptic endoscopy in head and neck and bronchial neoplasms has considerably improved the ease by which the diagnosis can be made.

CANCER SCREENING

There is now a very wide range of diagnostic techniques and screening procedures for the detection of cancer. In some centres it is possible for a patient to obtain a combination of the methods described above. For example, in addition to physical examination and blood investigations, routine chest x-ray, mammography, xeroradiography, thermography, cervical cytology (where appropriate), sigmoidoscopy and upper gastrointestinal endoscopy may be offered. As indicated previously, such a screening programme is not only expensive, but is time consuming for the patient. It is more normal for screening to be organised around specific organs. Thus cervical cytology or breast cancer screening may be offered to women. These examinations may be associated with other clinical examinations such as post-natal visits, or routinely at family planning clinics. In Japan, with a high incidence of gastric cancer, routine double contrast barium meal examinations and endoscopy may be offered.

Although it has been argued that the early diagnosis of most forms of cancer is associated with improved survival rates it remains important to consider the role of screening procedures in the early diagnosis of cancer. In breast cancer screening programmes using large populations of 'well-women' investigated with clinical or radiological methods, figures of between 1 in 100 and 1 in 1000 have been reported. One major study has been conducted to investigate the value of clinical examination and mammography in the reduction in mortality from breast cancer. Over 62 000 women from New York were involved and results showed that in the group of patients regularly screened, the mortality was reduced by one third. It is important to point out this reduction in mortality was *only* found in the over 50 age group. On the basis of this study, and several smaller trials, most would agree that screening of the over 50s with mammography may be a worthwhile procedure. In the under 50 age group only high risk patients and those with clinical indications should be screened.

In the case of cancer of the cervix it is now reasonable to conclude that regular cervical cytology has been associated with the reduction in mortality of the disease which has occurred in the past decade. The problem with cervical cancer is to screen the most appropriate population.

In Japan the routine use of endoscopy and radiology has resulted in the discovery of a high proportion of early lesions with a consequent reduction in the mortality.

The case for other forms of screening remains to be established. However, it is to be hoped that a combination of public education and effective screening techniques might result in a reduction in mortality.

24 Public Education on Cancer

Public education on cancer encompasses every form of communication which may affect the public's attitude to the disease. Thus education includes not only the information given to the public by doctors, and nurses, but by the media and lay personnel. The aim of public education is to ensure that the patient who suspects he might have cancer reports early to his primary care physician and is referred for appropriate therapy as soon as possible.

IS CANCER EDUCATION NECESSARY?

This is an important question. Any successful health education programme requires a dedicated band of workers, time and money. It is essential therefore that it can be justified. At the present time there are several compelling reasons for improving the state of knowledge the public has about cancer.

(1) Cancer is a common disease. As such it is a major public health problem affecting the whole community. Any factor which improved the early referral of patients would be of considerable importance.

(2) Many patients still present very late in the natural history of the disease. This may be due either to their own fear of the disease or to their inability to appreciate the signs or symptoms. Delay in presenting to the doctor may be due to many factors, including fear of the disease, fear of treatment or ignorance about current methods of cancer therapy. To see a young woman presenting with inoperable breast cancer which has been present for one to two years is perhaps reason enough for cancer education.

(3) There remains a great deal of ignorance about cancer itself. Many surveys have shown that most members of the lay public believe that cancer is the most common cause of death, that it is always associated with severe pain and suffering and that it can never be cured. These beliefs are, of course, unjustified but they do inhibit the early presentation of patients. In addition there are many 'old wives' tales about cancer, for example, it is often stated that cancer may be caused by knocks or blows, by 'bad living', or that it is related to 'moral degradation'. It is essential that such fears are dispelled.

(4) From what has been stated in an earlier section, it is clear that the earlier the cancer is treated the more favourable the outcome. Conversely when a patient presents with very advanced disease it is an extremely difficult problem to manage.

(5) Most patients are completely unaware of the many forms of treatment now available to the doctor treating cancer. They are often surprised that several methods can be used, often in conjunction with each other, and that the results of treatment are slowly improving.

Thus there are several reasons why education of the public should be pursued.

METHODS OF PUBLIC EDUCATION

Many methods are available, and they can be divided into two broad groups: methods used by non-medical personnel including the press, television and the teaching profession, and methods used by the medical and paramedical profession.

The Role of the Media

The use of the media is an extremely powerful method of reaching a large number of the public. Radio, television and the national press reach millions of people. Weekly magazines for women and the Sunday press are read by an enormous number of individuals. In general the articles produced and the programmes broadcast are of a high standard and are very informative. They often concentrate on the success aspects of cancer and deal with new methods of treatment and 'research breakthroughs'. Some articles, however, are appalling and present the problems in a way in which the individuals would not be encouraged to visit his or her doctor. So powerful are the media, however, that it becomes an important function of the profession as a whole to co-operate closely and supervise broadcasts or the publication of articles.

The Teaching Profession

As discussed later, one group which may be very amenable to education are school children. The teaching profession may therefore have an important role in health education, particularly in relation to smoking and hygiene.

Nurses and Health Visitors

This is a particularly appropriate group of professionals to be involved in cancer education. They are close to the patient, in touch with the relatives and know the home circumstances. They are able to carry out 'face to face' interviews and, when the occasion arises, to introduce such topics as smoking, cancer smear examinations or breast self-examinations. They are also able to note changes in the family and encourage early referral to the doctor. At a different level they may talk to young wives groups, or the elderly and use that opportunity to outline matters of health education.

The Medical Profession

The doctor carries a heavy responsibility for health education, and in his privileged position it is essential that he or she makes full use of the opportunity. The visit to the surgery with a cough or indigestion can be used to discuss problems of smoking or diet. The visit of a mother with an unwell child can be used to influence her about her own health. Again, at a different level, the doctor has a role in speaking to the public about cancer and to try, whenever possible, to present complex information in a way in which it is understandable to the public.

Obviously, it is necessary that professional education precedes public education. It is essential that the doctor or nurse is fully aware of recent advances in management and research in cancer. The back-up resources of experts in the area should be fully utilised. There is no doubt that the best educators are nurses, health visitors and doctors. They have the knowledge, the opportunity, and the skill to be used in advancing the public's knowledge about cancer. There is also no doubt that the fears of the doctor or nurse are the fears of the patient. If the doctor feels that there is no hope for treatment or that giving up smoking is not important then it is likely that the patient will hold the same views.

It is often considered that increasing education of the public will only increase the risk of developing 'cancerophobia'. There is no real evidence for or against this. The experience of most educators, however, is that to increase the awareness of the public to a health problem allows fears to be allayed rather than to increase them. There is also no doubt that cancer is a more dangerous disease than cancerophobia.

THE PUBLIC – WHICH GROUP SHOULD BE EDUCATED?

In an ideal world all individuals would have an equal opportunity to receive cancer education. With restricted resources, however, it is necessary to establish certain priorities. These may be related either to high risk groups or to groups whose potential for learning or whose motivation is greatest.

In the first category, as cancer incidence increases with age, one high risk group are the elderly. This group is often difficult to reach and to change opinions and beliefs. More use should be made of old folks clubs and pensioners social functions to improve education. Another group which can be fairly readily influenced is young married women following childbirth. The importance of regular cervical smears and breast self-examination can then be discussed.

One of the most receptive groups are schoolchildren, from the age of five upwards. This group has no preconceived notions of cancer, and if it can be gradually introduced in an appropriate way, many important aspects of health education can be taught. The concept of a 'non-smoking' generation begins in the school.

It should be obvious that there is no simple method of regularly contacting the group most at risk of developing cancer. It is essential, therefore, that no opportunity is lost in discussing cancer education with any patient who presents with any complaint no matter how trivial.

HEALTH EDUCATION OR CANCER EDUCATION?

It might have been assumed from the foregoing discussion that cancer education should be considered separately from health education. While it is essential that expertise is available in the field of cancer it is considered by most health educators that cancer education should be part of health education. This serves not only to integrate cancer education into a general plan of health education, but implies that cancer is not a separate, unique, untouchable disease, but that cancer is a word used for a whole group of diseases which require treatment and investigation just as any other illness. By integration it is hoped that some of the stigma associated with cancer will be diluted.

INFORMATION FOR THE PUBLIC

Having discussed the importance of cancer education and its role in improving the early referral rate of patients it is necessary to give some guide lines as to the kind of information required by the public. The following synoptic list gives some ideas for a health education programme.

The Basic Biology of Cancer

What is cancer? How does it start? These questions allow discussion on the nature of cancer and the fact that it is not a single disease but a whole group of diseases. It is possible then to describe the difference between normal cells and cancer cells and to mention the various forms of carcinogenesis. The differences between benign tumours and malignant tumours can be emphasised, and the problem of cancer spread in relation to early treatment detailed.

The Diagnosis and Treatment of Cancer

A simple outline of the various methods used for diagnosing cancer can be given. As far as treatment of cancer is concerned it is important to emphasise the multimodality approach to the problem and the fact that many different methods are now available. A discussion of the results of treatment of cancer comparing early treatment with treatment of patients with advanced disease can be given.

Warning Signs of Cancer

A question often asked is, how would I know I had cancer? This is a very difficult question since the signs and symptoms of cancer often mimic benign disease, and vice versa. A list of warning signs may be given but it is imperative that these are interpreted with caution. Any of the list given below may occur in benign disease and this fact *must* be emphasised. The presence of one of the signs noted below is an indication to see a doctor, not an indication of cancer.

(1) A lump in the breast or elsewhere.
(2) A sore that does not heal.
(3) Hoarseness or cough.
(4) Change in bowel or bladder habits.
(5) Abnormal bleeding vaginally or rectally.
(6) A mole that changes in size or colour.
(7) Indigestion or difficulty in swallowing.
(8) Unexplained loss of weight.

The Prevention of Cancer

It would be a gratifying achievement if simple rules for the prevention of cancer could be given. This, however, is not possible in the present state of knowledge and the following list simply documents some aspects of prevention which are already well known.

(1) When an abnormal sign or symptom occurs consult your doctor.
(2) Stop smoking cigarettes.
(3) Have a regular medical and dental check-up.
(4) Have a regular cervical smear.
(5) Practise regular breast self-examination.
(6) Avoid exposure to substances known to cause cancers, e.g. asbestos, chromates, etc.

It is hoped that as knowledge of cancer and its treatment progresses, this information will be passed on to the public in order that the best possible therapeutic results can be obtained in patients with the smallest amounts of tumour.

25 Terminal Care and Pain Control

Terminal care may be defined as the management of patients in whom the advent of death seems certain and not too far off, in whom the diagnosis has been accurately made and in whom care has turned from the curative to the palliative. Terminal illness, of course, is not specific to malignant disease. Yet cancer is often associated with death and dying, and with pain and suffering. It is for this reason that terminal care is discussed here.

To use the words terminal care is only one way of describing the situation and other terms such as continuing care, care of the dying, long-term care have been used. It is perhaps the finality of the words 'terminal care' which makes their use inappropriate.

From the rather simple definition given above several preliminary observations can be made about the nature of terminal care. First, the definition implies that the diagnosis has been accurately established. In a previous section the importance of 'sinister symptoms' in patients with malignant disease has been stressed. This is even more so in the terminal, or presumed, terminal illness. It may happen that patients are assumed to have terminal illness, when they may have treatable disease. It can be argued that investigation in such instances is unnecessary and indeed unethical. The following two case reports may illustrate the value of simple investigation.

A 45 year old married woman with breast cancer developed chest symptoms, including cough and breathlessness. It was assumed that these symptoms represented rapidly advancing disease and that she should be admitted to a terminal care home. She was treated with narcotic analgesia for almost a year, when the diagnosis was reviewed. Chest x-ray was clear, she was weaned off morphine and discharged. She required further treatment for recurrent breast cancer but at least was able to return home.

A 50 year old man with advanced gastric carcinoma developed cough and a pyrexia. The General Practitioner telephoned the hospital indicating that the patient was unwell and that he would look after him at home and make sure that he died comfortably. However, he was subsequently admitted, and chest x-ray showed chronic bronchitis. Following a course of antibiotics he was discharged home and he remained well for a further year.

These two anecdotes are used to illustrate the principle of diagnosis before the label terminal illness is given to any patient. This may not be easy, and indeed may be impossible. However, the few patients who benefit from this approach may justify its use.

The second point of the definition is that it is possible to know that death is certain and not too far off. It is an extraordinarily difficult thing to predict the time of death in patients with terminal illness. In such patients the time of death is related to the survival instinct of the patient, the symptomatology, the rapidity of progressing disease, and the presence of intercurrent problems such as infection. Yet the questions 'how long have I got to live?', or 'how long has my relative to live?' are common. No certain answer can be given and replies must be based on clinical experience and a knowledge of the individual patient.

The third point of the definition indicates clearly that in the patient with terminal illness care is turned on and not switched off. It is a very simple matter to neglect or forget about the patient with advancing disease. The hope of a miraculous cure has gone, heroic surgery, wonder drugs have no place, and the doctor may feel that he has nothing to offer, that he is inadequate. Yet this is the very time that the patient needs help and comfort and the support of the cancer care team. To look after patients with terminal illness is an active process. The more that is put into it, the more rewarding it becomes. How much easier it is to forget to visit the patient rather than to spend a little while at the bedside. It remains a difficult area; to talk to the young patient dying of cancer is not easy and emotional involvement in the family situation may place a heavy strain on any individual. Hence the importance of the cancer care team, and the ability of the members of the team not to show their fears and emotions. This is particularly the case with junior members of the medical and nursing profession who themselves may require the support of the team during the care of a patient dying with cancer.

THE AIMS OF TERMINAL CARE

What then are the aims of terminal care? Can a plan of action for their management be established? How best should symptoms be controlled? The aims of terminal care can be simply stated.

(1) The assessment and control of symptoms.
(2) The provision of an environment of caring.
(3) The provision of time to talk.

The two key words in management are 'assessment' and 'time': without an appreciation of their relevance the doctor will be unable to control symptoms effectively and to provide the patient with a death with dignity.

The four principles of management are as follows.

(1) Is the diagnosis correct? The importance of this has already been stressed.
(2) What are the main symptoms and how can they be controlled?
(3) Has conventional anticancer therapy been used to the full?
(4) What are the patients feelings? How is the family coping with the problem? Are there social problems which can be dealt with?

Clearly it is of major importance to assess and identify the symptoms which the patient has. This requires as thorough a clinical history and examination as would be performed in any patient. Thus a symptom such as 'back pain' may not be due to spinal metastases, but to urinary infection or constipation. Breathlessness may be related to congestive cardiac failure as well as to lung metastases. Does it matter what the symptom is due to? Does it really alter management? There is no doubt that breathlessness is a very distressing symptom. If due to heart failure then appropriate treatment may relieve symptoms and make the patient much more comfortable. It is unlikely that such treatment would significantly prolong life yet it might very significantly increase the comfort of the patient. Similarly the pain or frequency of a urinary infection may be readily relieved by antibiotics. It is stressed that such treatments are used specifically to treat symptoms and that non-symptomatic infectious disease in terminal illness may not necessarily be actively treated.

A common ethical problem is the use of intravenous fluids in such patients. Here, once again, it is symptomatology which is important. The patient with a dry mouth and parched throat unable to swallow will die more comfortably if fluids are given intravenously and meticulous attention given to mouth care.

During the assessment of symptoms consideration should always be given to conventional therapy. Even in terminal disease radiotherapy in small doses may readily relieve pain. Local toilet surgery may considerably improve the lot of a patient with an offensive ulcerating lesion.

The final problem is to assess the patient, his home and his family. The attitude of the patient is of considerable importance. The ability of the patient to cope with severe illness and physically distressing symptoms affects the psychological state of the individual. It is often the little things which bother patients most, hence the need for attention to the smallest details: the gardener, confined to bed, unable to see his flowers; the woman who because of pain or weakness is unable to knit; the reader, unable to concentrate long enough to read a few pages. Such relatively small things become magnified in the minds of patients and require careful and thoughtful handling.

The attitude of the family is also important. They must be made to feel part of the care effort. They will require support and comfort, and may also require social or financial assistance: the young mother with children struggling to hospital to see her husband; the elderly woman, determined to keep her husband at home; the breadwinner not wishing to lose his job, yet anxious to do all he can to visit or care for his wife. Such problems are not uncommon yet they only come to light after a careful history has been taken and the relatives interviewed. In the appendix a list of agencies which may help the patient and his relatives is given.

One of the aims of terminal care is the provision of an environment of caring. This is a rather trite phrase and within old hospital buildings or difficult home circumstances it may be an impossible end to achieve. The meaning of this aim is that the patient, in whatever circumstances he may be, home or hospital, is made to feel that someone cares. It is so easy in hospital to relegate the terminally ill to the distant corners of the ward. Yet if the patient is alert, the company and fellowship of other patients must not be shunned. Such patients should be brought into the companionship of the ward rather than excluded. It is particularly appropriate that the medical staff still visit the patient regularly, indeed more often than usual. To sit by the bedside for a few moments, to hold the patient's hand, or pass a few minutes in conversation makes a world of difference to the patient. Nursing staff too have a special responsibility in making the caring environment seem real.

The final aim of terminal care follows naturally from the above, the provision of time to talk and sit with the patient. Doctors and nurses are always in a hurry. Hospital wards are busy places, often noisy and full of people who rush past not caring or having the time to care. Even at home the routine of the family life must go on, and it must seem to patients that no one has any time to stop, and sit and listen. It may not be for a long time, a few moments will often suffice, but the fact that someone has stopped and listened can work wonders. It is during such moments that the patient's real feelings, anxieties and frustrations often become apparent. Small things come to light which can usually be rectified, but would not have been heard of without time being taken.

To the young doctor or nurse the thought of talking to a dying patient is often terrifying. They feel that they will be unable to cope with the difficult questions which might be asked or that their own emotional involvement in the problem will be too great. There is no way in which such conversations can be made simple or easy, yet it is surprising how well one can cope when faced with difficult problems.

THE SYMPTOMS OF TERMINAL ILLNESS

Because of the very wide spectrum of malignant disease, the symptomatology associated with terminal illness is very varied indeed. The approach outlined above, assessment and diagnosis and a general medical approach to the problem is the only way in which symptoms can be readily, and rapidly, relieved. Pain is the symptom most usually associated with cancer yet it is much less common than supposed. Pain will be dealt with separately later.

Before considering specific symptoms it is pertinent to mention the question of prevention of serious and distressing complaints. These involve attention to nursing care particularly related to skin and mouth. Thus good nursing can prevent bed sores and the excoriation which may occur with incontinent patients. Regular mouth hygiene will prevent a dry mouth with sore tongue and cracked lips. Daily baths, unless the patient is severely incapacitated, also maintains cleanliness and allows full inspection of the skin. The patient should be encouraged to sit out of bed and walk wherever possible.

Mouth Problems

Regular mouth hygiene with chlorhexidine washes may take care of ulceration or soreness. Regular inspection and the use of locally active antifungal agents, where appropriate, may relieve symptoms of pain. Frequent small sips of water, juice or ice may relieve the dry mouth.

Anorexia

This is a very common symptom of advanced malignant disease. It is often very difficult to control. The use of corticosteroids, such as Prednisolone, 5 mg three to four times daily, may improve appetite. Some anabolic steroids, such as nandrolone phenylpropionate may also be of benefit. The use of alcohol, such as a glass of sherry, before meals may stimulate appetite.

Nausea and Vomiting

When the vomiting is of an obstructive nature the use of strong analgesics and anti-emetics may relieve colic-like symptoms. When the obstruction is high up in the gastrointestinal tract the use of a nasogastric tube with suction may be preferable to heavy sedation.

When nausea is a major problem with or without vomiting various anti-emetics including metoclopramide, cyclizine, prochlorperazine or chlorpromazine may be used. Regular medication is often essential.

Constipation

This symptom may be related to the presence of tumour or secondary to the use of analgesics. Where possible regular mild aperients are best and Milpar or liquid paraffin may be sufficient. Where the problem is more severe an initial enema followed by the use of locally active suppositories may be necessary. When the patient is still able to swallow and has no intestinal obstruction, the use of a high roughage diet may be sufficient to ensure regular bowel action.

Diarrhoea

This may be related to the tumour, secondary to the use of drugs, related to infection or to an impacted rectum. Simple rectal examination and rectal swab for bacteriological analysis will allow exclusion of the two latter. Where diarrhoea or rectal discharge is tumour related, the use of codeine phosphate, 15–60 mg three times a day, or Lomotil, two to three tablets daily, may control this symptom. When this is accompanied by severe pain morphine or one of its derivatives may act in a dual manner.

Following upper gastrointestinal operations with by-pass procedures, diarrhoea may be related to a blind-loop syndrome, the failure to re-absorb bile acids or to pancreatic insufficiency. In these cases the use of antibiotics, cholestyramine or pancreatic replacement therapy, respectively, may be required.

Dysphagia

This is an extremely troublesome symptom. Not only may the patient have pain and be unable to take food, but he may have problems with swallowing his own saliva with consequent choking and dyspnoea. When this occurs adequate sedation is necessary.

Hiccough

This may be associated with diaphragmatic irritation or with a metabolic cause such as renal failure. It may be controlled by the use of metoclopramide or chlorpromazine.

Ascites

Recurrent ascites may cause dyspnoea and pain. Where possible regular paracentesis should be performed. In the terminal phase there is little place for the instillation of chemotherapeutic agents, radioactive isotopes or radiotherapy.

Cough

This may be related to tumour or to infection. When severe, control of the infection with antibiotics may be justified. Control with methadone syrup 5–10 ml, or Benylin expectorant, may be sufficient. Where pain is also a problem Diamorphine will also relieve cough. When the sputum is thick Bromhexine, 8 mg three times a day, will often allow the patient to cough more easily.

Dyspnoea

Dyspnoea is a particularly troublesome symptom as it may be associated with anxiety. The symptom itself may be caused by primary or secondary malignant disease in the chest, pleural effusion, cardiac failure, intra-abdominal pressure or chest infection. The dyspnoea may be associated with bronchospasm. Where possible any intra-abdominal problem such as ascites should be dealt with and pleural effusion tapped. Where cardiac failure is present this is treated with diuretics and Digoxin. A bronchodilator such as Salbutamol, 2–4 mg three times a day, or aminophylline suppositories may be indicated. Where a large amount of tumour is present Prednisolone may be helpful, as will opiates. Where anxiety is present the use of Diazepam may be necessary. If the dyspnoea is related to infection there may be a case for using antibiotics specifically to relieve symptoms. When a distressing rattle is present on breathing, hyoscine 0.4–0.6 mg intramuscularly may prevent the accumulation of secretions. When dyspnoea occurs suddenly, as with a pulmonary embolus, the use of opiates and hyosine will rapidly relieve symptoms.

Urinary Frequency

This may be caused by tumour growth, previous therapy such as radiation, surgery or chemotherapy, or related to infection. When the urine is infected the use of the appropriate antibiotic should help. With other problems the use of Emepronium bromide, 100 mg three times daily, may be of use. When the symptoms are severe catheterisation may be required. This should be carried out using strict asceptic precautions. Regular bladder washouts with hibitane or noxyflex may be necessary.

Pruritus

With increasing jaundice or skin involvement with tumour, pruritus may be a problem. Cholestyramine may be indicated where there is obstructive jaundice. Antihistamines or steroids may be necessary when other conditions are present.

Insomnia

This is a frequent complaint of patients and, therefore, it is necessary to ask about it specifically. Non-barbiturate sedatives are preferred – dichloral-phenazone or nitrazepam. In the elderly chlormethiazole may be helpful but it is always important to remember that confusion may easily result from the use of such drugs.

Confusion

It is important to exclude a metabolic cause for this including renal failure, hypercalcaemia or abnormal electrolyte levels. Prednisolone may be very useful in the patient with a raised serum calcium. When ectopic hormones such as antidiuretic hormones are being released fluid restriction may help. Confusion may also be related to an infection and, if severe, antibiotics may be indicated. Other causes of confusion may be treated symptomatically with chlorpromazine, diazepam or thioridazine.

Anxiety and Depression

Not surprisingly these symptoms may be present in patients with terminal illness. In great measure they may be relieved by attention to other physical and psychological problems of the patient. When necessary the use of diazepam in anxiety and the tricyclic antidepressants such as amitryptiline may be required.

Local Skin Problems

Fungating lesions on the skin may be particularly distressing to the patient. The smell may be offensive and the wound itself associated with pain. Regular dressings with eusol and a topical antibiotic cream may reduce the local problem. Even in the terminal phase, consideration should be given to tumour specific therapy.

PAIN CONTROL IN TERMINAL ILLNESS

It is often assumed that patients with cancer will experience severe pain at some time in their illness. This is not the case. In most series only 15–20 per cent of patients with cancer have severe pain. Even in specialist units dealing with patients with terminal illness only 60–65 per cent of patients will have a major pain problem. In such patients the majority will experience complete relief of pain. This achievement has been related to the development of certain principles of pain control.

(1) The diagnosis of the cause of the pain. This has been emphasised already.

(2) An understanding of the nature of chronic pain. This type of pain, and the methods required for control, are unlike those for acute pain. Chronic pain is present continuously and gradually increases in intensity. It wears the individual down by being constantly in his mind. Other feelings or thoughts are often unable to be considered because of pain. Trivial complaints are often exaggerated because of pain and the patiently urgently requires relief.

(3) The importance of regular therapy. Because chronic pain is present all the time, the only way to abolish it effectively is by the use of regular analgesia. Pain should be anticipated and the next dose of drug timed to be given before pain starts again. With chronic pain related to cancer there is little place for drugs to be given 'as required' or 'PRN'. If this is done the pain may return, the patient asks for analgesia and before the drug has time to be effective the pain has become severe again. Regular therapy, then, is the basis of pain control, the timing and the dosage being adjusted to meet the needs of the individual patient.

(4) Explanation to the patient. It is important to the patient to know what treatment is being given and why. He may be informed that to achieve the

correct dosage will take time. During this period it is essential that the patient is closely observed, his reactions noted, and the severity of pain and the level of control achieved recorded. If the dosage is insufficient, then it should be increased. Dose escalation, modification of the drug used and changes in the timing of the drug may all be required.

(5) Addiction is not a problem in terminal illness. It is surprising how many clinicians still hold back treatment by opiates because of the fear of addiction. In patients with only a few days or weeks to live it is unlikely that addiction would be a problem. If large doses of narcotic analgesia are required, as is frequently the case, the dosage can often be reduced once effective pain control is achieved. In a similar way, the respiratory depression associated with such drugs is of little clinical significance.

METHODS OF PAIN CONTROL IN THE PATIENT WITH CANCER

There are now many methods available for controlling pain in the cancer patient. They can be broadly divided into two groups: those which are specifically directed at the tumour responsible for the pain and those directed at general or local pain control.

Radiotherapy

Even in terminal illness effective pain control may be achieved by the use of radiotherapy. Bone pain and pain related to locally invasive tumour may be treated by a short (1–5 day) intensive course of radiotherapy, or even by a single treatment.

Chemotherapy

Even in advanced disease chemotherapy may significantly alleviate pain. The choice of drugs and the dosage schedule will depend considerably on the type of tumour.

Drug Therapy in the Control of Pain

Analgesic therapy is often the simplest method of pain control. Successful therapy depends on adequate dosage, regularly given. Titration of the patient's pain against the dosage of the drug is the basis of therapy.

It is usually worthwhile starting with a mild analgesic given regularly. Soluble aspirin or Paracetamol are the usual drugs and it is surprising how many patients respond to this simple form of therapy. When patients have obviously had severe pain it is often worthwhile starting with a stronger drug.

For moderate pain the use of dipipanone with cyclizine (Diconal) given as

1–2 tablets four hourly is often effective. Dihydrocodeine (DF118) is not as effective but is an extremely useful drug. Phenazocine (Narphen) or Pentazocine (Fortral) may also be used.

When severe pain is present it is necessary to use the narcotic analgesics. Whenever possible these should be given orally. Diamorphine and cocaine elixir is the most useful. This is made up in various strengths with additives such as prochlorperazine or chlorpromazine. Because of the many different formulations it is important not to prescribe 'Brompton's mixture', rather a specific prescription should be used and adhered to. The diamorphine and cocaine elixir BPC should be used more often. Morphine or pethidine may also be used. Methadone is another potent drug but since it has a longer duration of action overdosage of the patient should be watched for.

The above guide lines form the basis of treatment. Individual modifications may be required, such as the use of aspirin or phenylbutazone in the treatment of pain which has an inflammatory basis. With the wide range of preparations available there is little excuse for inadequate pain control in the majority of cases.

Neurosurgical Methods of Pain Relief

Numerous methods are now available ranging from local nerve blocks to cordotomy. Such methods are often successful in achieving excellent pain control. Local nerve blocks, such as the injection of alcohol or phenol into an intercostal nerve may rapidly relieve bone pain in the rib cage. Various forms of intrathecal injections, e.g. hypertonic saline or phenol, may ablate lower limb or pelvic pain. Cordotomy performed surgically or percutaneously by electrical techniques or methods for the alteration of thalamic function have also been used. The above techniques, in experienced hands, are very safe and give excellent pain control. They should be used in conjunction with the other methods described.

Because of the wide range of expertise required in the treatment of pain there is a case for the development of pain groups or pain clinics where the experience of several specialities – neurosurgeons, anaesthetists, radiotherapists, physicians and pharmacologists – can be gathered together.

TERMINAL CARE IN CHILDHOOD

This presents the cancer care team with one of its most difficult clinical problems. There are inevitable tensions on the professional side as well as with the relatives. Emotional attachments formed during the period of care may make the terminal phase of the illness particularly traumatic. The child in the meantime remains in the middle, conscious of the strains. Children, particularly of school age and above, may have a concept of death which is different to that of adults. They see it not associated with pain or suffering, but as a form of separation which may not seem as final as it does in adulthood. They may talk about death in a more material way than adults and accept it as inevitable but this does not lessen the load. Children in general do not like lies and they are often more astute than appreciated. Special expertise and experience are required in dealing with dying children.

TERMINAL CARE: A SUMMARY

The care of the patient with terminal illness differs little from that of a patient with any other form of disease. The same skill and care are required. The patient requires to be treated as an individual with self-respect and dignity. The care of the patient with cancer, and the philosophy of the clinician, is well summed up in the following quotation:

Guerir quelquefois:	Cure sometimes
Soulager souvant:	Give relief often
Consoler toujours:	Comfort always

26 The Logistics of Cancer Care

Cancer is a high incidence disease. As such it is essential that the individual patient with cancer is given the most appropriate therapy in an environment most suited to his own needs. It is important therefore to consider the organisation of cancer services. The organisation should take into account the following aspects.

(1) A large number of patients are involved.

(2) A wide variety of medical specialists are concerned with the treatment of cancer and patients may be referred in many ways.

(3) The general practitioner or primary care physician should be involved in the care of the patient.

(4) It is likely that community services, such as district nursing facilities or ambulances may be required. It is important, therefore, to consider the location of hospital treatment in relation to this.

(5) Any organisation must take into account developmental aspects of cancer management and be closely associated with teaching of undergraduate, postgraduate and paramedical personnel.

Bearing in mind these points, there are several ways in which cancer care has been organised. The undermentioned methods have been used in several countries and are not necessarily mutually exclusive.

Current practice in the United Kingdom. At the present time referral patterns to individual consultants produces an acceptable clinical service. Most patients are handled efficiently, are given up-to-date treatment by the most appropriate specialist, and, as the patient is usually referred locally there can be integration of community facilities and general practitioner care. More specialised regional services such as radiotherapy can be provided accordingly. The deficiency of this method is that development and teaching are often given a low priority.

The comprehensive cancer centre or the cancer hospital. This has definite advantages. Such institutions are centres of excellence, composed of a number of specialists with particular expertise in management or in investigative procedures. Patients are treated to a high standard and development and teaching form an integral part of such a service. The disadvantages are that no matter how large the hospital is, it is unlikely that all patients can be treated in the centre. In addition, patients may be removed a considerable distance from home, family and friends.

Small, highly specialised units, dealing with relatively rare forms of cancer, or developmental units dealing with particular tumour types. Such organisations have had considerable success in advancing knowledge of particular forms of cancer, notably the leukaemias and lymphomas. There is a case for centralising the treatment of other forms of cancer which have a low incidence in order to make the best use of resources and to gain the most experience. Such tumours, in addition to those mentioned above, might include eye tumours, bone tumours, thyroid neoplasms and the melanomas. With the more prevalent solid tumours such as breast, lung or gastrointestinal cancers, the developmental or investigative group has a very definite place. It should be realised that it is unlikely that all tumours even of a single type could be treated in such a unit.

Specialised units of cancer medicine with district hospitals or teaching hospitals. Such units, co-ordinated and integrated closely with the individual specialists within the hospital, provide an advisory service and encourage teaching and research. They have the advantage of being within district hospitals and so retain the patient close to the referring consultant and allow the patient to stay close to his home environment, family, community services and general practitioner.

The four options outlined above are only a few of the possible ways of organising a cancer service. Which method (or methods) chosen will depend on the individual circumstances of the area and its particular requirements. It should be remembered, however, that if newer methods of treatment are to be employed, particularly the use of chemotherapy or immunotherapy, then increasing resources in terms of out-patient space, day-bed facilities, paramedical and medical personnel will be required. It has been said that Hodgkin's disease was an easy disease to treat before it was treatable. The fact that effective therapy became available meant that patients required more in-patient and out-patient care, they required to be reviewed regularly and they used an increasing amount of investigative time. With a relatively rare form of cancer such improvements in treatment can usually be accommodated by expanding existing services. However, if a more effective form of therapy for carcinoma of lung became available then it might drain existing resources very considerably if that therapy required any additional facilities. These facts should be considered in the organisation of cancer services.

Organisational aspects of clinical practice are often accorded a low priority by many doctors. Yet in the field of cancer care simple changes in the organisation of services might result in improved care for a fairly high percentage of the population.

Appendix: Help Agencies in Cancer Care in the United Kingdom

(1) Department of Health and Social Security grants, attendance allowances.

(2) Local authorities, meals on wheels, district nurses, health visitors, night nursing. Provision of aids (e.g. commodes). Social work departments. Domicillary nursing.

(3) Local societies, e.g. Samaritans, provide funds from endowments. The hospital Social Work Service will advise.

(4) Marie Curie Foundation Homes, Homes Department, 138 Sloane Street, London, SW1X 9AY.

(5) Hospice care. A number of hospices for terminal care operate in all regions.

(6) Red Cross. Local Red Cross branches give assistance and provide aids.

(7) National Society for Cancer Relief, Michael Sobell House, 30 Dorset Square, London, NW1.

(8) Malcolm Sargent Fund for Children, Chief Administrator, 56 Redcliffe Square, London, SW10.

(9) Ileostomy Association of Great Britain and Ireland, 149 Harley Street, London, W1N 2DE.

(10) Mastectomy Association, 1 Colworth Road, Croydon, CR0 7AD, Surrey.

(11) Tenovus Cancer Information Centre, 111 Cathedral Road, Cardiff, CF1 9PH.

Bibliography

Bagshawe, K. D. (1975). *Medical Oncology*, Blackwell Scientific Publications, Oxford

Becker, F. F. (Ed.) (1975). *Cancer I: A Comprehensive Treatise*, Plenum Press, New York and London

Currie, G. A. (1974). *Cancer and the Immune Response*, Current Topics in Immunology, Edward Arnold, London

Greenspan, E. M. (1975). *Clinical Cancer Chemotherapy*, Raven Press, New York

Greenwald, E. S. (1973). *Cancer Chemotherapy*, Henry Kimpton, London

Holland, J. F. and Frei, E. III (Eds.) (1974). *Cancer Medicine*, Lea and Febiger, Philadelphia

International Union Against Cancer (1973). *Clinical Oncology. A Manual For Students and Doctors*, Springer-Verlag, Berlin

Saunders, C. (1978). *Management of Terminal Malignant Disease*, Edward Arnold, London

Schottenfeld, D. (Ed.) (1975). *Cancer Epidemiology and Prevention*, Thomas, Springfield, Illinois

Symington, T. and Carter, R. L. (1976). *Scientific Foundations of Oncology*, Heinemann Medical Books, London

Tooze, J. (Ed.) (1973). *The Molecular Biology of Tumour Viruses*, Cold Spring Harbor Laboratory

Walter, J. (1973). *Cancer and Radiotherapy*, Churchill–Livingstone, Edinburgh and London

Walter, J. and Miller, H. (1969). *A Short Textbook of Radiotherapy*, Churchill–Livingstone, Edinburgh and London

Index